Electrotherapy

with Model Answers

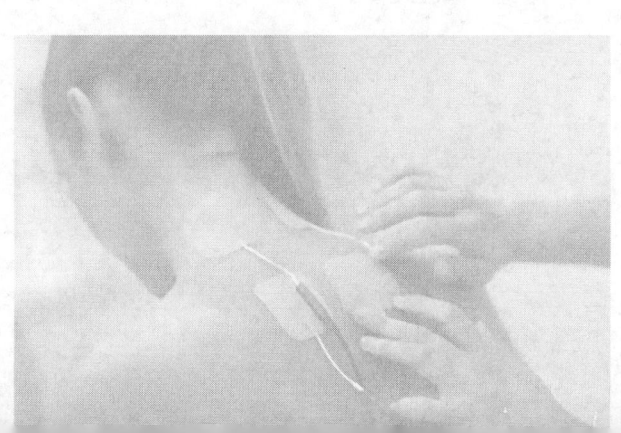

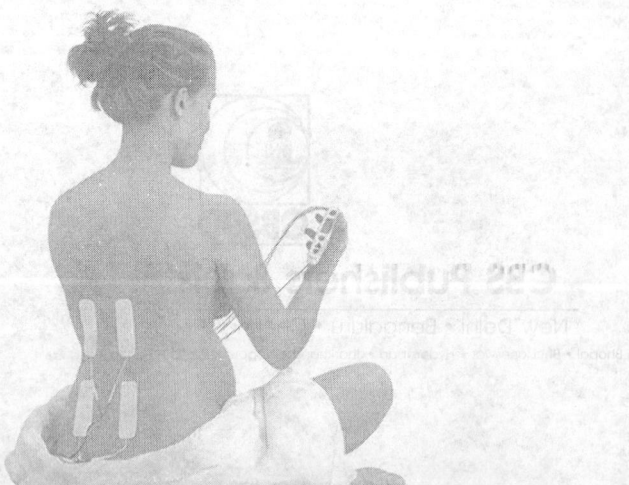

Electrotherapy

with Model Answers

Shyam Devidas Ganvir MPTh, PhD (MUHS)
Professor and Principal
DVVPFS College of Physiotherapy
Ahmednagar, Maharashtra

Nitin Suhas Nikhade MPTh
Professor
Maharashtra Academy of Engineering Education and Research (MAEER's)
Physiotherapy College, Talegaon Dabhade, Pune, Maharashtra

Amit Vinayak Nagrale MPTh, PhD (Scholar)
Associate Professor
Maharashtra Institute of Physiotherapy
MIMSR Medical College, Latur, Maharashtra

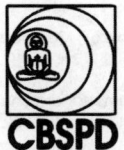

CBSPD

CBS Publishers & Distributors Pvt Ltd

New Delhi • Bengaluru • Chennai • Kochi • Kolkata • Mumbai

Bhopal • Bhubaneswar • Hyderabad • Jharkhand • Nagpur • Patna • Pune • Uttarakhand • Dhaka (Bangladesh)

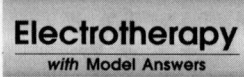

Electrotherapy
with Model Answers

ISBN: 978-93-88327-58-9

Copyright © Authors and Publisher

First Edition: 2019

Reprint: 2025

Published by Satish Kumar Jain and produced by Varun Jain for

CBS Publishers & Distributors Pvt Ltd

4819/XI Prahlad Street, 24 Ansari Road, Daryaganj, New Delhi 110 002, India
Ph: 011-23289259, 23266838   Website: www.cbspd.com
e-mail: delhi@cbspd.com

Corporate Office: 204 FIE, Industrial Area, Patparganj, Delhi 110 092

Ph: 011-4934 4934   Fax: 011-4934 4935   e-mail: publishing@cbspd.com; publicity@cbspd.com

Branches

- **Bengaluru:** Seema House 2975, 17th Cross, K.R. Road, Banasankari 2nd Stage, Bengaluru 560 070, Karnataka, India
  Ph: +91-80-26771678/79   Fax: +91-80-26771680   e-mail: bangalore@cbspd.com
- **Chennai:** 18/8B, Subbarayan Street, Shenoy Nagar, Chennai 600 030, Tamil Nadu, India
  Ph: +91-44-42032115, 26681266   e-mail: chennai@cbspd.com
- **Kochi:** 42/1325, 1326, Power House Road, Opp KSEB, Kochi, 682 018, Kerala, India
  Ph: +91-484-4059061-67   Fax: +91-484-4059065   e-mail: kochi@cbspd.com
- **Kolkata:** 147, Hind Ceramics Compound, 1st Floor, Nilgunj Road, Belghoria, Kolkata 700 056, West Bengal, India
  Ph: +91-33-25633055/56   e-mail: kolkata@cbspd.com
- **Lucknow:** Basement, Khushnuma Complex, 7-Meerabai Marg (behind Jawahar Bhawan), Lucknow 226 001, Uttar Pradesh, India
  Ph: +91-522-4000032   e-mail: tiwari.lucknow@cbspd.com
- **Mumbai:** PWD Shed, Gala no. 25/26, Ramchandra Bhatt Marg, Next to JJ Hospital Gate no. 2, Opp. Union Bank of India, Noorbaug, Mumbai 400 009, Maharashtra, India
  Ph: +91-22-66661880/89   e-mail: mumbai@cbspd.com

Representatives

• **Hyderabad**	0-9885175004	• **Jharkhand**	0-9811541605	• **Nagpur**	0-8692091830
• **Patna**	0-9334159340	• **Pune**	0-9664372571	• **Uttarakhand**	0-9716462459

Printed at Glorious offset, Delhi, India

Preface

While teaching classes on electrotherapy, we were frequently asked by our students, "Is there a book we would like to recommend which includes the model answers that cover all the information?" and we would respond, "One of these days, we will write one." So, when we were invited by CBS Publishers & Distributors to frame a text, we immediately nodded our heads.

Presently, there is lack of books on model answers in electrotherapy; we believe none covers the information within the same breadth and depth as this one. In writing this book, we tried to meet the need that we believed existed—the need for a book on model answers in electrotherapy that covers the breadth and depth of this material in a readily accessible and easy to understand manner. We have simulated the questions and answers in such a way that leads the reader to conceptualize the subject and imitate their thoughts in the scientifically sound and appropriate manner.

After reading this book, the reader will be familiar with all the physical agents used by rehabilitation clinicians, including thermal agents, water, mechanical agents, and electrical agents. The reader will also understand the types of patient problems that can be treated effectively with physical agents and the physical properties and physiological effects of physical agents. It is designed to provide students/learners with the opportunity to experience each of the physical agents first hand, ask and answer pertinent questions regarding their application, and explore patient scenarios to help foster a greater comfort level and understanding. This book provides rehabilitation students and practising therapists with thorough understanding and firm basis for applying electrical agents in rehabilitation.

This book includes twelve chapters. Chapter 1 recalls the physics principles and laws of electricity. Details about fundamentals of low frequency currents including production of electricity, mains supply, types of AC/DC currents are provided. It describes the various types of electrodes used in therapeutics, electrical skin resistance and significance of various media used to reduce skin resistance. The information is presented first so that information gained can be used for selection and application of physical agents.

In Chapter 2 the reader learns about the fundamentals of high frequency currents which include types of transformers, EMF, semiconductors and electronic circuit oscillators. Chapter 3 deals with electromagnetic spectrum and laws of transmission. Chapter 4 explains the cellular physics while environmental and man made electromagnetic field at the cellular level and risk factors on prolonged exposure are being covered in Chapter 5.

Chapter 6 covers the physical and physiological bases of physical agents including production, physical principles, panel diagram and testing of apparatus. It also provides information on electromagnetic agents, including ultrasound, interferential therapy, ultraviolet, lasers, and diathermy that apply electro-magnetic radiation to achieve therapeutic effects.

Chapter 7 integrates various types of DC currents and their waveforms. Chapter 8 highlights various types, basis concepts and production of medium frequency currents. Chapter 9 justifies about principles, types and production of various high frequency physical therapy modalities. Chapter 10 reveals about various modalities used for actinotherapy. Chapter 11 mentions principle and method of application, and physiological effects of various superficial heating agents. Chapter 12 describes methods of testing of different physical therapy modalities.

This is the book on electrotherapy that we and our students have been looking for. The logical and consistent format of each chapter makes the presented information readily accessible, and the depth of information facilitates the reader's understanding of how physical agents may be applied safely and effectively to enhance patient rehabilitation and succeed in examinations.

Shyam Devidas Ganvir
Nitin Suhas Nikhade
Amit Vinayak Nagrale

Acknowledgments

The authors take this opportunity to gratefuly acknowledge the assistance and contribution of the few veterans who had faith in this undertaking.

We bestowed and bow our head to almighty God and our beloved parents to whom we owe as they are the medium due to which we are able to contribute to the society in the scientific manner.

Deserving of special mention Dr GJ Ramteke, the living legend, and well known figure in the field of physiotherapy fraternity, who has always been a source of inspiration for this book. We were fortunate to have him as our faculty and guide for the answering the questions related to electrotherapy subject in the appropriate and methodological format. He has taught us the various ways which we wanted to share with the student for their upgradation of knowledge. We acknowledge the publishers for considering and taking this work ahead for the sake of welfare of the students and, last but not the least, our beloved I and II BPTh students who motivated us for the providing us an insight for doing something for them.

Shyam Devidas Ganvir
Nitin Suhas Nikhade
Amit Vinayak Nagrale

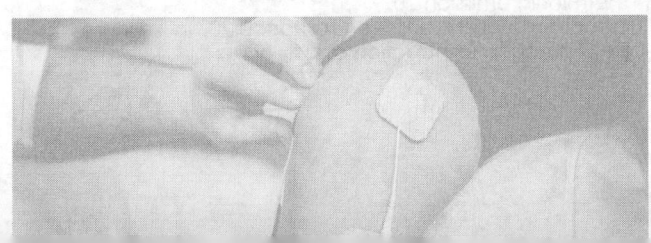

Contents

Basic Physics

SHORT ANSWER QUESTIONS

Structure of Atom (3 Marks)

An atom is defined as the smallest particle of an element, which may or may not have an independent existence.

It can be described as having a central nucleus, surrounded by a cloud of electrons revolving in a definite orbit. Modern research reveals that an atom is further composed of subatomic particles. These are electrons, protons and neutrons (Fig. 1.1).

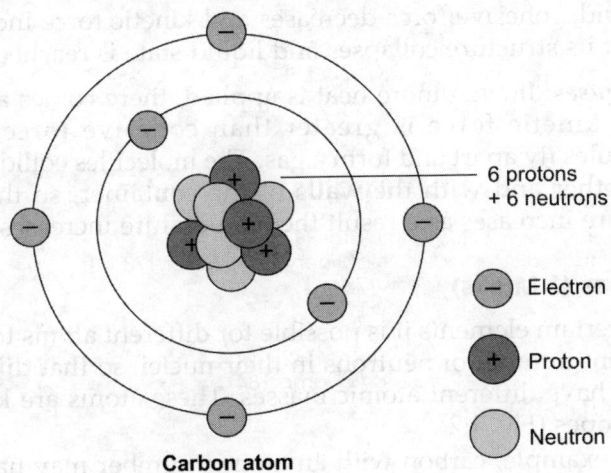

6 protons
+ 6 neutrons

— Electron

+ Proton

Neutron

Carbon atom

Fig. 1.1: Bohr's atomic model of a carbon atom

1

Proton: This is comparatively large nuclear particles which possess a positive charge exactly opposite to the negative charge of an electron.

Neutron: This is a nuclear particle with a mass almost equal to that of a proton, but is electrically neutral, i.e. neither positive nor negative.

Electrons: They are negatively charged particles found revolving in orbit around the nucleus and in the neutral atom their number equals the number of protons.

States of Matter (3 Marks)

Matter: It is defined as anything that has mass and occupies space.

Matter exists in any one of the three states, viz. solid, liquid and gases.

The state of matter is dependent upon temperature, pressure and its own nature.

In solids: There is a strong cohesive force which holds them in a rigid lattice formation so that shape remains same or constant. The kinetic force produces vibrations of molecules about a mean position.

In liquids: When considerable amount of energy is applied to liquid, cohesive force decreases and kinetic force increases so that its structure collapses and liquid state is reached.

In gases: If even more heat is applied, there comes a point when kinetic force is greater than cohesive force; then molecules fly apart and form a gas. The molecules collide with each other and with the walls of the container, so that the pressure increases as a result the temperature increases.

Isotopes (3 Marks)

With certain elements it is possible for different atoms to have different number of neutrons in their nuclei, so that different atoms have different atomic masses. These atoms are known as isotopes (Fig. 1.2).

For example, carbon with an atomic number may have an atomic mass of 12, 13, or 14, these atoms having 6, 7 and

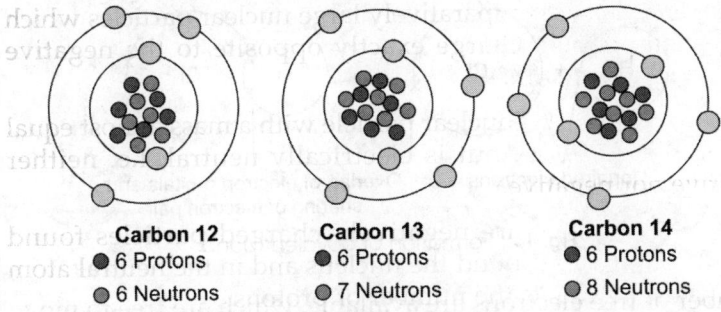

Carbon 12
● 6 Protons
● 6 Neutrons

Carbon 13
● 6 Protons
● 7 Neutrons

Carbon 14
● 6 Protons
● 8 Neutrons

Fig. 1.2: Isotopes of carbon

8 neurons, respectively. An isotope is an atom of an element which contains the standard number of protons but a non-standard number of neutrons.

Ionic and Covalent Bonds (3 Marks)

An ionic bond is formed when an atom of one element gives an electron to the atom of another element, the first one becoming a positive ion, the second one becoming a negative ion. These atoms are then held together by their opposite electrical charges, since unlike charges attract. For example, common salt or sodium chloride (Na^+Cl^-) (Fig. 1.3).

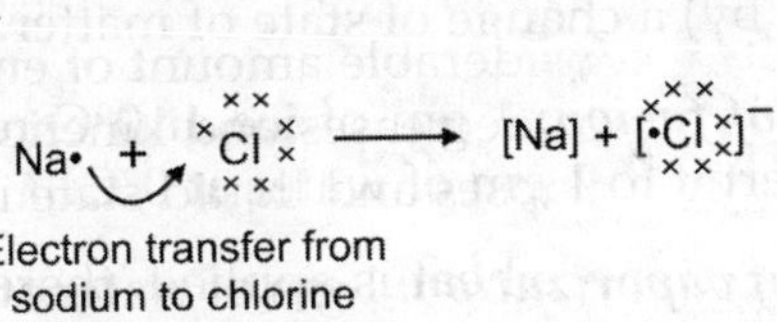

$$Na\cdot + \overset{\times\ \times}{\underset{\times\ \times}{\times}Cl\times} \longrightarrow [Na] + [\overset{\times\ \times}{\underset{\times}{\cdot}Cl\times}]^-$$

Electron transfer from
sodium to chlorine

Fig. 1.3: Formation of ionic bond

A covalent bond is formed when the outer shells of the atoms of the elements share a number of common or bonding electrons so that, in effect each atom has a complete outer shell (Fig. 1.4). For example, a covalent bond (HCl) is formed between hydrogen and chlorine by sharing a pair of electrons.

Conductors and Insulators (3 Marks)

Conductors: These are the substances that easily allow the flow of electric charge through them. In such substances a large

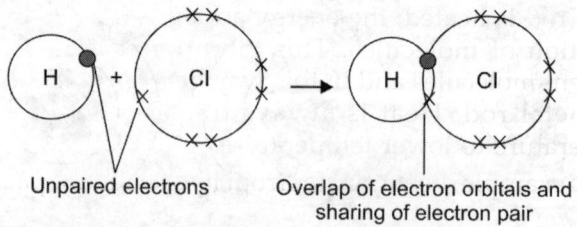

Unpaired electrons   Overlap of electron orbitals and
sharing of electron pair

Fig. 1.4: Formation of covalent bond

number of free electrons are available, which are free to move about in the whole conductor.

Examples, copper, aluminium, iron, etc.

Insulators: These are the substances that do not allow the flow of electric charge through them. They have negligibly small number of free electrons.

Examples, glass, rubber, wood, etc.

Latent Heat (3 Marks)

A specific amount of energy is required to change the solid form of a particular substance into a liquid or the liquid into a gas. This energy is called *latent heat* and is the energy required for (or released by) a change of state of matter.

Latent heat of fusion: 1 gm of ice at 0°C requires 336 J of energy to convert it to 1 gm of water at 0°C.

Latent heat of vaporization: 1 gm of water at 100°C requires 2268 of energy to convert it to 1 gm of steam at 100°C.

Practical application: Ice melting on the skin takes considerable energy (heat) from the skin, thus cooling it, whereas paraffin wax solidifying on the skin gives out considerable heat to the skin, thus warming it.

Transmission of Heat (3 Marks)

There are three mechanisms of transmission of heat:

1. *Conduction:* The transfer of heat by conduction requires physical contact between the two objects or heat transfer from one point to another within a body. If one end of solid

metal rod is heated, the energy added causes an increased vibration of molecules. This vibration is transmitted to adjacent molecules and in this way heat is conducted along the metal rod. Heat is always transferred from higher temperature to lower temperature.

For example, heat transfer from hydrocollator pack to the skin.

2. *Convection:* It takes place in a circulating liquid or gas. If one part of the fluid is heated, the kinetic energy of the molecules in that part is increased, they move further apart and this part becomes less dense. Consequently it rises, displacing the more dense fluid above which descends to take its place. The currents so produced are called *convection currents.*

For example, transfer of heat from one part to other parts of the body through blood circulation.

3. *Radiation:* Heat may be transmitted by infrared electro-magnetic radiation through space without any intervening matter or movement. The heating of certain atoms causes an electron to move to a higher energy electron shell. As it returns to its normal shell, the energy is released as a pulse of infrared electromagnetic energy.

For example, IR lamp emits infrared radiations that cause heating of the tissues.

Physical Effects of Heat (7 Marks)

1. *Rise in temperature:* The average kinetic energy of constituent molecules increases.

2. *Expansion of the material:* Increased kinetic energy due to heating of an object produces a greater vibration of molecules, which move further apart and expand the material. Gases will expand more than the liquids and liquids more than solids.

3. *Change in physical state:* Heat may cause a solid to change into a liquid and a liquid into a gas. Changing a substance from one physical state to another requires a specific amount of heat energy (i.e. latent heat) without raising the temperature.

4. *Acceleration of chemical reaction:* van't Hoff's law states that any chemical reaction capable of being accelerated is accelerated by a rise in temperature.

5. *Production of an electrical potential difference:* If the junction of two dissimilar metals (e.g. copper and antimony) is heated, a difference of potential is produced between their free ends. Conversely, an electromotive force (EMF) applied to the junction of two metals can cause a rise in temperature at the junction.

6. *Production of electromagnetic waves:* When energy is added to an atom (by heating), an electron may move out into a higher-energy electron shell. When the electron returns to its original shell, energy is released as a pulse of electromagnetic waves.

7. *Thermionic emission:* Heating of some materials like tungsten may cause such molecular agitation that some electrons leave their atoms and may break free of the metal. This leaves a positive charge which tends to attract electrons back. A point is reached where the rate of loss of electrons equals the rate of return, and a cloud of electrons then exists as a space charge around the metal. This process is known as thermionic emission.

8. *Reduction in viscosity of fluids:* Dynamic viscosity is the property of fluid (liquid or gas) offering internal friction between the two adjacent layers. The molecules in the viscous fluid are quite strongly attracted to one another. Heating increases the kinetic movement of these molecules, reducing their cohesive mutual attraction and making the fluid less viscous.

Electromagnetic Radiation (3 Marks)

Electromagnetic (EM) radiation is a form of energy propagated through free space or through a material medium in the form of electromagnetic waves, such as radio waves, visible light, and gamma rays.

EM radiation is so-named because it has electric and magnetic fields that simultaneously oscillate in planes mutually perpendicular to each other and to the direction of propagation through space.

Electromagnetic radiation is produced by the movement of electrons within the atom. If energy is added to an atom, e.g. by heat, this can cause an electron to move out to a higher-energy electron shell (excited state). When the electron returns to its normal level, energy is released as a pulse of electromagnetic energy (a photon).

General Properties of Electromagnetic Radiation (3 Marks)

1. Electromagnetic radiation can travel through vacuum. Does not need a medium to be transmitted unlike mechanical waves in water or sound waves in air.
2. Electromagnetic radiation travels through space at speed of light. The speed of light is always a constant.
3. Electromagnetic radiation has the dual nature; it exhibits wave properties and particulate (photon) properties.
4. Wavelengths are measured between the distances of either crests or troughs. It is usually denoted by the Greek symbol λ. Entire band of energies is grouped in the electromagnetic spectrum.

Static Electricity

SHORT ANSWER QUESTIONS

Static Electricity (3 Marks)

When the charges on the body do not flow then it is called static electricity.

The simplest way of producing a static electric charge is to rub two insulators, such as glass and flannel; a positive charge is produced on the flannel and a negative charge on the glass.

This is because electrons are transferred from the superficial atom of flannel to the surface of glass. The charges are held on the surfaces of the objects and spread themselves evenly over the surface, unless there are points and corners, where the charges tend to concentrates.

Characteristics of Charged Body (7 Marks)

1. **Distribution of the charge:** The electric charge is always held on the surface of the object.

   The charge tends to concentrate where the curvature of the surface is greatest. It spreads evenly over a sphere (Fig. 2.1a) but concentrates at the edges and corners of a flat plate (Fig. 2.2b).

2. **Behavior of like and unlike charges:** Two electrically charged objects exert a force on one another, called electrostatic force. Like charges repel and unlike charges attract each other due to electrostatic force (Fig. 2.2).

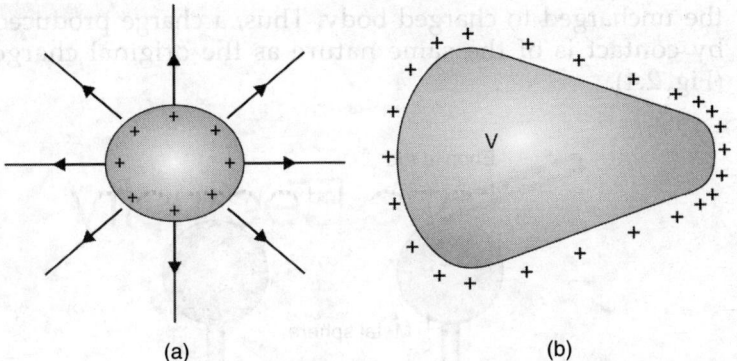

Fig. 2.1a and b: Distribution of electric charges on the surface of the object

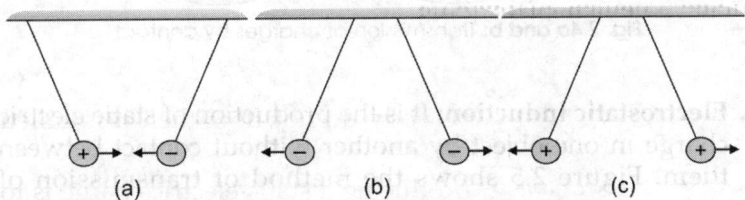

Fig. 2.2a and b: Like charges repel and unlike charges attract each other

3. **Transmission of electric charge:** It is possible to transfer electric charge from one object to another. Usually electrons are transferred, and the body that gains electrons acquires an excess of negative charge. The body that loses electrons has an excess of positive charge (Fig. 2.3).

   When an object with a positive charge makes contact with one which is electrically neutral, some electrons pass from

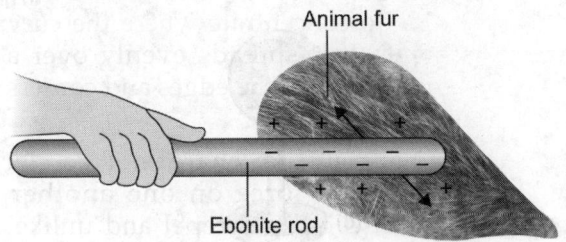

Animal fur

Ebonite rod

Fig. 2.3: Transmission of electric charge

the uncharged to charged body. Thus, a charge produced by contact is of the same nature as the original charge (Fig. 2.4).

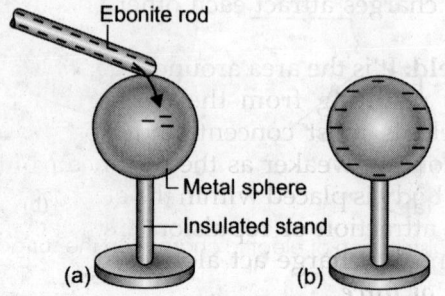

(a) (b)

Fig. 2.4a and b: Transmission of charges by contact

4. **Electrostatic induction:** It is the production of static electric charge in one object by another without contact between them. Figure 2.5 shows the method of transmission of charges by electrostatic induction.

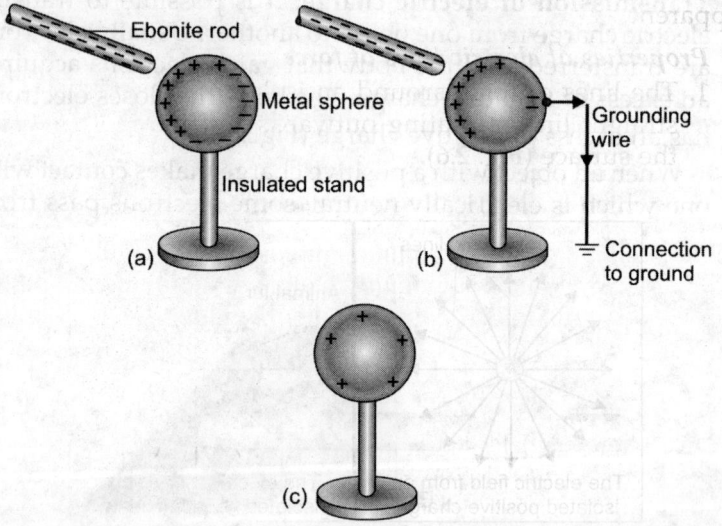

(a) (b)

(c)

Fig. 2.5a to c: Transmission of charges by electrostatic induction

5. **Attraction for light objects:** A charged object attracts an uncharged body which, if sufficiently light, moves towards it. The charged object induces a charge of the opposite type on the adjacent surface of the uncharged one, the unlike charges attract each other and the objects move together.

6. **Electric field:** It is the area around a charged body in which the forces resulting from the charge are apparent. The electric field is most concentrated closed to the charged object, becoming weaker as the distance from it increases.

When one body is placed within the electric field of another, the forces of attraction or repulsion are effective. The forces resulting from the charge act along definite lines known as *electric lines of force.*

Properties of Electric Lines of Force (7 Marks)

Electric lines of force: The forces resulting from the charge act along definite lines, known as *electric lines of force.* These are the lines along which a free negative charge would move if placed within the electric field.

Electric field: The electric field is an area around a charged body in which the forces resulting from the charge are apparent.

Properties of electric lines of force

1. The lines of force around an isolated charged body are straight lines radiating outwards and perpendicular to the surface (Fig. 2.6).

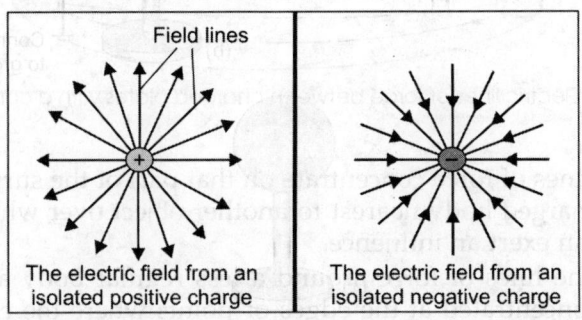

Field lines

The electric field from an isolated positive charge

The electric field from an isolated negative charge

Fig. 2.6: Electric field around an isolated charged body

2. Lines of force are considered to travel from positive to negative.
3. Between two objects with opposite charges the lines of force pass from one to the other, but spread out somewhat, as they tend to repel each other (Fig. 2.7).

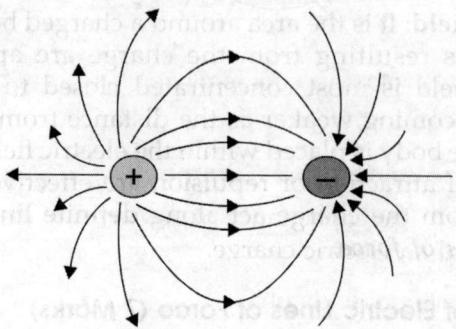

Fig. 2.7: Electric field between oppositely charged object

1. Lines of force pass readily through conductors and less through insulators. If a conductor, such as a metal sphere is placed within the field, the lines of force concentrate on it because they can pass through it easily (Fig. 2.8).

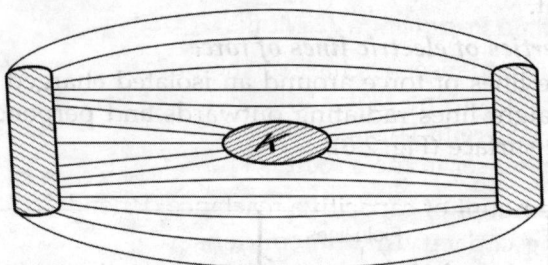

Fig. 2.8: Electric lines of force between charged plates with a conductor in the field

2. Lines of force concentrate on that part of the surface of a charged body nearest to another object over which they can exert an influence.
3. The lines of force around a less regular body are most concentrated at the edges or points where the charge is concentrated (Fig. 2.9).

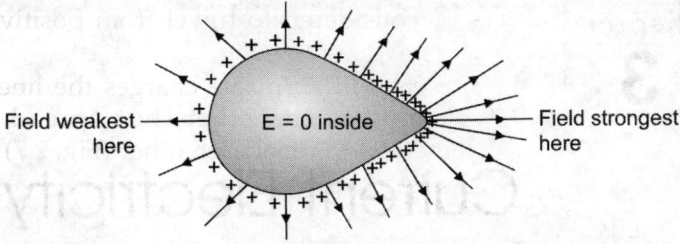

Fig. 2.9: Electric field and charge distribution around a pear-shaped conductor

Capacitance and its Unit (Summer 2017) (3 Marks)

Capacitance: The capacitance of an object is the ability of the body to hold an electric charge.

Capacitance depends on:
- Material of the body
- Surface area of the body

There is an inverse relationship between capacitance and potential.

Unit of capacitance is farad (F) but practically micro-farad is used.

Capacitive Reactance (3 Marks)

When a condenser is charged the potential difference developed between the plates offers increasing impedance to the charging current. This impedance offered to the flow of current by a condenser in the circuit is known as *capacitive reactance*.

The amount of capacitive reactance depends on:
1. The capacity of the condenser, with which it varies inversely.
2. The frequency of the current, as higher the frequency the less is the impedance.

Current Electricity

SHORT ANSWER QUESTIONS

Current Electricity (3 Marks)

An electric current occurs when there is flow of charged particles (electrons) in a conductor. By historical convention, conventional current always flow from positive to negative which is opposite to the flow of the electrons.

Electrons will flow only for as long as the potential difference and a conducting pathway exist. It is of two types:

Direct current: The electric current whose direction does not change with time whether its magnitude changed or not is called direct current.

Alternating current: Electric current whose magnitude and direction both changes with time periodically are called alternating current.

Theories of Electricity (3 Marks)

The electron theory: It is based on the fact that every object consists of a very large number of atoms, each of which normally has an equal number of protons and electrons. The opposite charges balance each other and the object is electrically neutral. A generator of electricity causes disturbance of the electrons and the object either gains electron, becoming negatively charged or loses electron, becoming positively charged.

If a connection is made between two objects, one with negative and other with positive charge, electrons pass from the former to the latter until the charges are equalized. This flow of electrons constitutes an electric current, which according to the electron theory, passes from negative to positive.

The one fluid theory: This theory postulated that electricity was an invisible and weightless fluid, present on all objects but capable of being disturbed. If the fluid was at the normal level the object was electrically neutral, but an increase in the quantity of fluid gave rise to a positive charge and a decrease to a negative charge.

If a connection was made between two oppositely charged objects fluid passed from the positively charged object to that with a negative charge, constituting an electric current. The one fluid theory has now been supressed by the electron theory. But it explains the diversity of custom in tracing electric currents.

AC and DC Currents (3 Marks)

The rate of flow of electric charge through a conductor is called electric current. It is of two types:

Direct current: The electric current whose direction does not change with time whether its magnitude changed or not is called direct current (Fig. 3.1).

Alternating current: Electric current whose magnitude and direction both changes with time periodically are called alternating current (Fig. 3.2).

An electric current is AC or DC depending on the voltage source connected with the given circuit.

Potential Difference (3 Marks)

The electrical potential of a body is the electrical condition of that body when compared to the neutral potential of the earth. Bodies with an excess of electrons are called negative and bodies deficient in electrons are called positive.

A difference of potential exists between similar bodies charged with different quantities of electricity. If a conducting

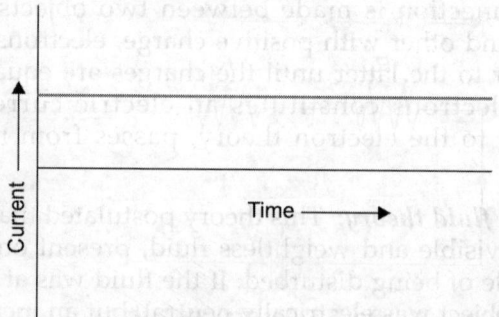

Fig. 3.1: Direct current

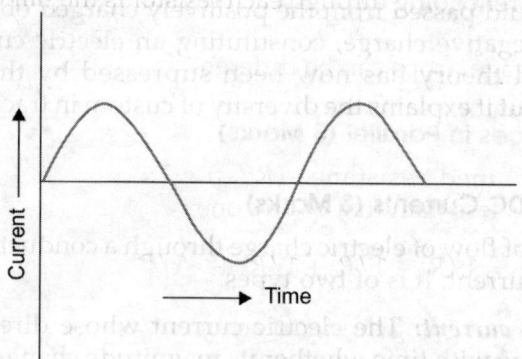

Fig. 3.2: Alternating current

connection is made between the two bodies, electrons will flow from the more negative body to the less negative one. Electron flow continues until both objects are at the same potential.

The force producing the movement of electrons is called an electromotive force (EMF). The greater the potential difference, the greater the EMF. Both are measured in volts.

Resistances in Series (3 Marks)

If resistances are connected in series, the total resistance equals the sum of individual resistances (Fig. 3.3).

$$R_{total} = R_1 + R_2 + R_3 + \dots R_n$$

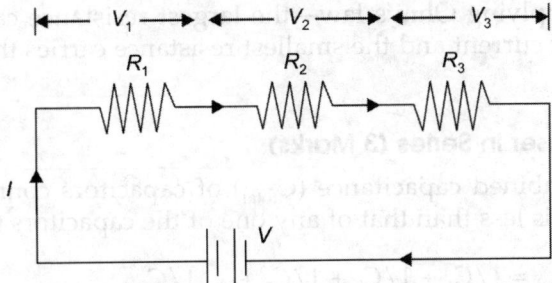

Fig. 3.3: Resistances in series

- Current going through each resistor is the same and equal to I.
- Voltage drops can be different; they sum to V.

Resistances in Parallel (3 Marks)

The combined resistance (R_{total}) of resistors connected in parallel is less than that of any one of the resistors (Fig. 3.4).

$$1/R_{total} = 1/R_1 + 1/R_2 + 1/R_3 + ... 1/R_n$$

- Current going through each resistor can be different; they sum to I.
- Each voltage drop is identical and equal to V.

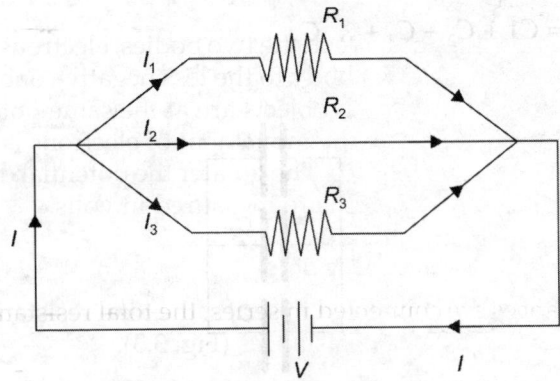

Fig. 3.4: Resistances in parallel

By applying Ohm's law—the largest resistance carries the smallest current and the smallest resistance carries the largest current.

Condenser in Series (3 Marks)

The combined capacitance (C_{total}) of capacitors connected in parallel is less than that of any one of the capacitors (Fig. 3.5).

$$1/C_{total} = 1/C_1 + 1/C_2 + 1/C_3 + \dots 1/C_n$$

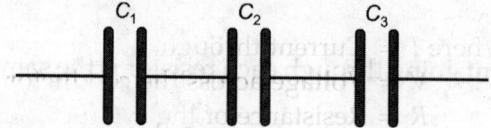

Fig. 3.5: Condenser in series

- Current going through each capacitor is the same and equal ($I_{total} = I_1 = I_2$).
- Voltage drops can be different for each capacitor ($V_{total} = V_1 + V_2$).

Condenser in Parallel (3 Marks)

If condensers are connected in parallel, the total capacitance equals to the sum of individual capacitors (Fig. 3.6).

$$C_{total} = C1 + C_2 + C_3 + \dots C_n$$

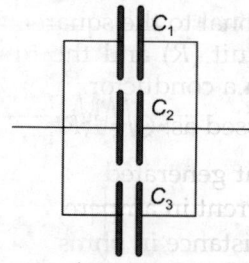

Fig. 3.6: Condenser in series

- Current going through each capacitor can be different $(I_{total} = I_1 + I_2)$.
- Voltage is same for each capacitor $(V_{total} = V_1 = V_2)$

Ohm's Law and Joule's Law (3 Marks)

Ohm's law: It states that provided the physical conditions (temperature, pressure, strain on conductor, etc.) remain constant, the current flowing through conductor is always directly proportional to the potential difference across its two ends and inversely proportional to resistance of the circuit.

$I = V/R$

> Where I = Current through a conductor (amperes)
> V = Voltage across the conductor (volts)
> R = Resistance of the conductor (ohm)

Joule's law: It states that the heat produced in the conductor after passing current through the wire is directly proportional to the square of the intensity of current, electrical resistance of the conductor and the time for which electric current passes through the conductor.

$Q = I^2Rt$ where Q = Heat generated in a conductor
> I = Current through a conductor (amperes)
> R = Resistance of the circuit (ohm)
> t = Time for which current flows (sec)

Thermal Effect of Electric Current (3 Marks)

The amount of heat produced when passage of electric current through a conductor can be calculated using *Joule's law*, which states that, the amount of heat produced in the conductor is proportional to the square of the current (I^2), the resistance of the circuit (R) and the time (t) for which the current flows through a conductor.

This may be expressed as: $Q = I^2Rt$

> Where Q = Heat generated
> I = Current in ampere
> R = Resistance in ohms
> t = Time in seconds

The mechanism of heat production can be explained on the basis of electron theory, which states that, when a potential difference is applied across conductor, an electric field is established at each point and hence electrons are accelerated in opposite direction. These electrons collide with the positive ions and lose their energy. The energy dissipated is changed into heat energy. In physiotherapy department, the devices like SWD, MWD, ultrasound, UVR, IRR, etc. are based on thermal effect of electric current.

Thermionic Emission (3 Marks)

The heating of molecules of some materials, e.g. tungsten, may cause molecular agitation that some electrons leave their atoms and may even break free of the surface of the metal. This leaves a positive charge on the atom which tends to attract the negative electrons back. However, a point is reached where the rate of loss of electrons exceeds the rate of return and a cloud of electrons then exists as a space charge around the object. The process is called thermionic emission and this is the principle upon which electric valves (diode and triode) work.

Inductance (3 Marks)

It is the ability of the conductor to have an EMF induced in it. Inductance depends on:

- The number of turns of wire present in the coil
- The proximity of the turns of wire to each other
- Whether or not there is an iron core present to concentrate the magnetic field.

Unit of inductance is Henries.

Inductive Reactance (3 Marks)

The "back" EMF produced by self-induction opposes the rise in intensity of current. This impedance to the flow of current in the circuit resulting from the self-induced EMF is known as inductive reactance.

The amount of impedance from inductive reactance depends on the strength of the self-induced EMF which is determined by:

1. The inductance of the conductor, with which it varies directly.
2. The rate of change in intensity of the current flowing in the conductor. The greater the rate of change the greater is the self-induced EMF.

Note: There is no inductive reactance with a constant DC.

Electromagnetic Induction and its Types (7 Marks)

Electromagnetic induction is the means by which electricity is produced from magnetism (vice versa). It is the result of interaction between a conductor and magnetic lines of force.

An EMF is produced in the conductor by magnetic lines of force surrounding a magnet, without contact with each other, but it is necessary for one to move relative to the other.

Three factors for electromagnetic induction are:

1. A conductor
2. Magnetic lines of force
3. Relative movement of 1 and 2

If the conductor is part of closed circuit, magnetic lines of force produce an EMF which causes movement of the electrons in the conductor. This can be shown by ammeter across the coil of wire.

Types of electromagnetic induction are: Mutual induction and self-induction.

1. *Mutual induction*: When an EMF is induced in an adjacent conductor by the magnetic field set up around a coil of wire carrying varying current, the process is known as mutual induction (Fig. 3.7).
2. *Self-induction:* When a current flows through a coil of wire, it sets up magnetic lines of force around each turn of wire. If the current varies in intensity these magnetic lines of force cut across turns of wire and induce an EMF in that same conductor, the process is known as self-induction.

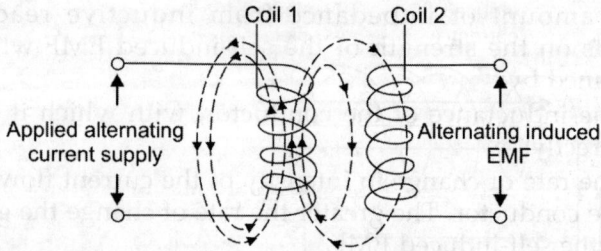

Fig. 3.7: Mutual induction of EMF

When primary current increases, magnetic lines of force move out, cutting adjacent turns of wire and thus inducing an EMF in them. The direction of induced EMF will be opposite to the force producing it (Lenz's law). The induced EMF is in the opposite direction to primary current and so opposes its rise. Self-induced EMF of this type is called *backward EMF* (Fig. 3.8a and b).

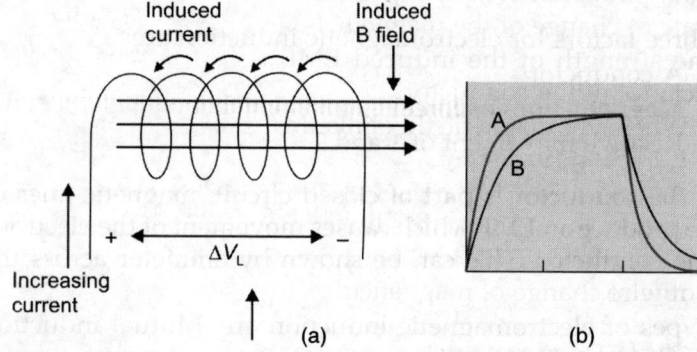

Fig. 3.8a and b: (a) Direction of self-induced EMF when current is rising; (b) Magnetic (B) field

When primary current starts to fall magnetic field is collapsed and line of force move back in, cutting adjacent turns of wire but in opposite direction than before. Induced EMF is also in opposite direction and flows forward as a *forward EMF* (Fig. 3.9a and b).

Lenz's and Faraday's Laws (3 Marks)

Lenz's law: It states that the *direction of the induced EMF* is such that it tends to oppose the force producing it.

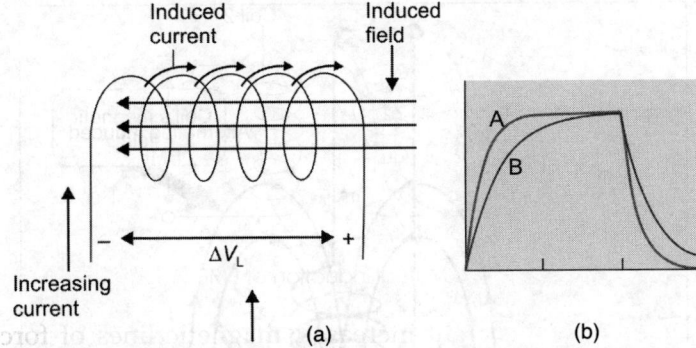

Fig. 3.9a and b: Direction of self-induced EMF when current is falling

For example, when the current in the primary coil is rising in intensity the EMF induced in the secondary coil is in the opposite direction to that applied to the primary.

Faraday's law: Faraday's law of electromagnetic induction states that the *strength of the induced EMF* is proportional to the rate of change of the magnetic field.

The strength of the induced EMF is proportional to the inductance of the conductor.

1. Whenever magnetic flux linked with a circuit changes an EMF is induced in it.
2. An induced EMF exists in the circuit, so long as the change in magnetic flux linked with it continues.
3. The induced EMF is directly proportional to the negative rate of change of magnetic flux linked with the circuit.

Eddy Currents (3 Marks)

- Any conductor lying in a varying magnetic field has an EMF induced in it. If the conductor is solid piece of material, magnetic lines of force passing through it set up circular currents at right angles to the magnetic lines of force are known as **eddy currents** (Fig. 3.10).
- Eddy currents are perpendicular to the magnetic lines of force and produce heating effect in tissues in accordance with Joule's law.
- In Fig. 3.10, a solid conductor is present in the varying magnetic field which produces the eddy currents in it,

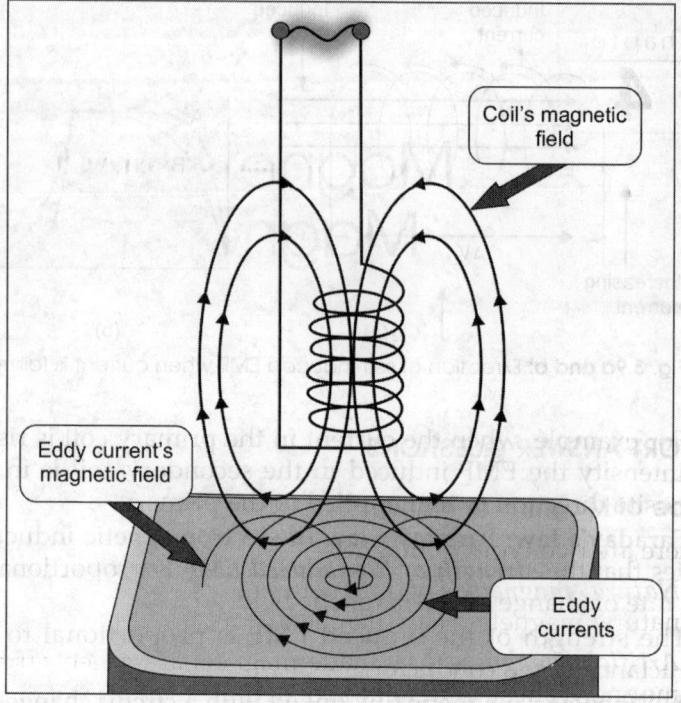

Fig. 3.10: Eddy currents

shown by arrows, whose direction is opposite to the magnetic lines of force which produce it. These currents are greatest near the surface of the conductor.

- In many electrical apparatus eddy currents are unwanted and are prevented by laminating the conductor. However, eddy currents are used to produce heat in the patient's tissue, in the inductothermy method of SWD.

Magnets and Magnetism

SHORT ANSWER QUESTIONS

Type of Magnets (3 Marks)

There are two types of magnets:

1. *Natural magnets:* The magnets found in nature are called natural magnets. These magnets are weak and shapeless.

2. *Artificial magnets:* Manmade magnets are called artificial magnet. These magnets are strong and have different shapes. They may be bar-shaped, horseshoe shaped, magnetic needles, magnetic compass, etc.

Types of artificial magnets

1. *Temporary magnets:* Magnetism of these magnets is temporary. It is made of soft iron.

2. *Permanent magnets:* Magnetism of these magnets is permanent. It is made up of steel, nickel and cobalt.

Magnetic Poles (3 Marks)

Magnet: A piece of substance which possesses the property of attracting small pieces of iron towards it is called a magnet.

The points inside the magnet, where attraction is maximum are called poles of magnet. Every magnet has two poles, viz. north pole and south pole.

A freely suspended magnet sets itself in the direction of geographic north and south.

North pole: End of the magnet pointing towards north is called north seeking pole or north pole.

South pole: End of the magnet pointing towards south is called south seeking pole or south pole.

Electromagnet (3 Marks)

An electromagnet consists of a coil of wire wound onto a soft iron bar (Fig. 4.1). When a current passes through a coil of wire it magnetizes the bar by induction. This is called an *electromagnetism*.

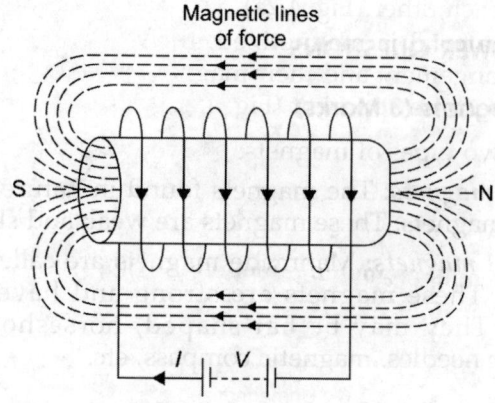

Fig. 4.1: Electromagnet

Wire carrying an electric current produce magnetic field around a straight wire in the form of concentric circles with the wire at their center. The magnetic field produced reinforces that of the coil and the resultant field is very strong. As soon as the current is put off, the magnetic effect is lost. The direction of magnetic lines of forces is given by right hand thumb rule.

Properties of Magnet (3 Marks)

1. A freely suspended magnet sets itself in the direction of north to south. If displaced from this direction it again returns to its original position.
2. Similar poles repel and opposite poles attract each other.

3. A magnetic field is the area or zone of influence around a magnet in which its magnetic force is apparent. The field is made up of magnetic lines of forces.

Molecular Theory of Magnetism (3 Marks)

If a magnet is broken in two, each part forms a complete magnet, however often the process is repeated. It is, therefore, assumed that the individual molecules of the magnetizable materials are tiny magnets. Their magnetic properties result from the rotation of electrons in their orbits.

When material is not magnetized, the molecular magnets lie in a haphazard manner and their magnetic properties neutralize each other (Fig. 4.2a).

When material is magnetized, the molecules assume an orderly arrangement and their magnetic effects augment each other and become apparent (Fig. 4.2b).

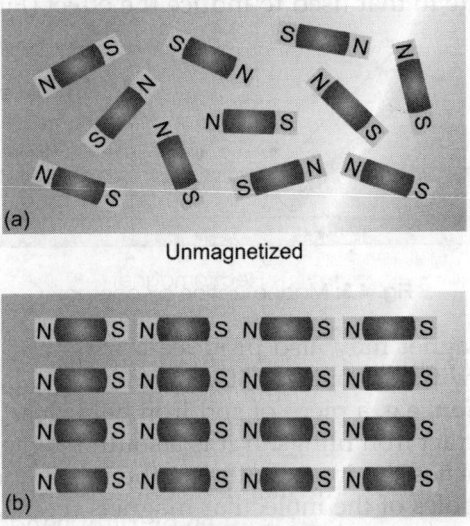

(a)

Unmagnetized

(b)

Magnetized

Fig. 4.2a and b: Arrangement of molecules in a piece of magnetic material

Properties of Magnet (7 Marks)

Magnet: A piece of substance which possesses the property of attracting small pieces of iron towards it is called a magnet.

Magnet possesses following properties:

1. **Setting in a north-south direction:** As the earth itself is a giant magnet; the earth's magnetic field will influence a suspended magnet. A freely suspended magnet sets itself in the direction of north to south. If displaced from this direction it again returns to its original position.

2. **Like magnetic poles repel one another:** North repels north and south repels south. Unlike magnetic poles attract one another.

3. **Isolation of poles:** Isolated north or south pole is not possible.

4. **Transmission of properties:** A magnet can produce properties of magnetism in suitable materials. As one pole of a bar magnet is stroked along the material, all the opposite poles of the molecular magnets are attracted towards it so that the object is magnetized.

   The end that the magnet leaves will have the pole opposite to that used to induce the effect (Fig. 4.3).

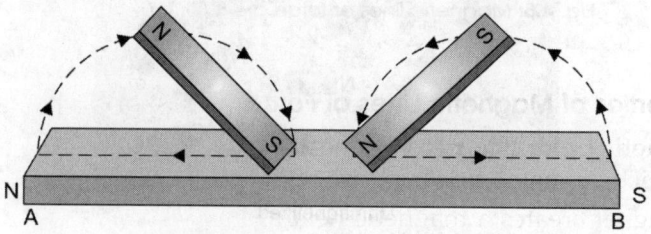

Fig. 4.3: Magnetization by contact

A magnet may also produce a magnetic effect in an object without contact between them is called *magnetic induction,* e.g. a piece of soft iron held close to a magnet will attract iron filings. If it is a south magnetic pole that approaches the iron, it attracts the north and repels the south poles of the molecular magnets (Fig. 4.4).

5. **Attraction of suitable materials:** Magnets attract certain materials. This effect is produced by magnetic induction.

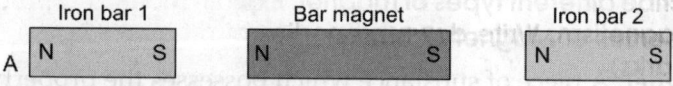

Fig. 4.4: Magnetization without contact (magnetic induction)

6. A magnetic field: This is the area or zone of influence around a magnet in which its magnetic forces are apparent. The field is made up of magnetic lines of force (Fig. 4.5).

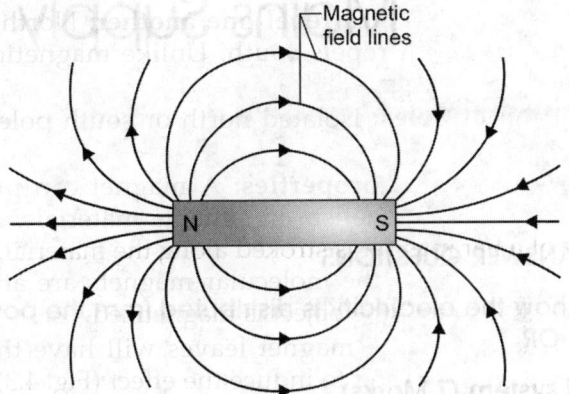

Fig. 4.5: Magnetic lines of force around a magnet

Properties of Magnetic Lines of Force (3 Marks)

Magnetic field: The area or zone of influence around a magnet in which its magnetic forces are apparent (Fig. 4.5).

Magnet creates a magnetic field around them. This field is being made up of *magnetic lines of force* which have the following properties:

1. They travel from north to south, which is the path a free north pole would take.
2. They attempt to take the shortest route possible but repel one another so that they infact become curved.
3. They travel more easily through some materials, e.g. magnetizable metals, than through others.

Describe different types of magnet. Explain molecular theory of magnetism. Write down properties of magnet (5 + 3 + 7 = 15 Marks)

Same as above answers.

Mains Supply

SHORT ANSWER QUESTIONS

Explain how the electricity is distributed from the power station? OR

The grid system (7 Marks)

Distribution of electricity: Current for mains supply is produced by dynamos at power stations. The current generated in the power station is supplied to the consumer by one live wire and one neutral wire, so the current is not earth-free. The cables may be carried across country by pylon, or in towns, taken underground enclosed in thick layers of insulation. The electricity is supplied throughout the greater part of the country by means of grid system.

Grid system: This is a system by which the electricity supplies throughout the greater part of the country are linked together. The supply is AC at 240 volts and a frequency of 50 cycles per second.

A three-phase current is used for distribution. Each dynamo has three coils of wire which follow each other through the magnetic field so that a separate current is generated in each coil. One end of each coil is connected to a live distribution line while the other ends are connected together and to earth. Distribution of current is by three live cables, one from each of the dynamo coils, and one neutral cable, which is common to the three live wires (Fig. 5.1). These four cables can be observed on the pylons which carry the cables across country.

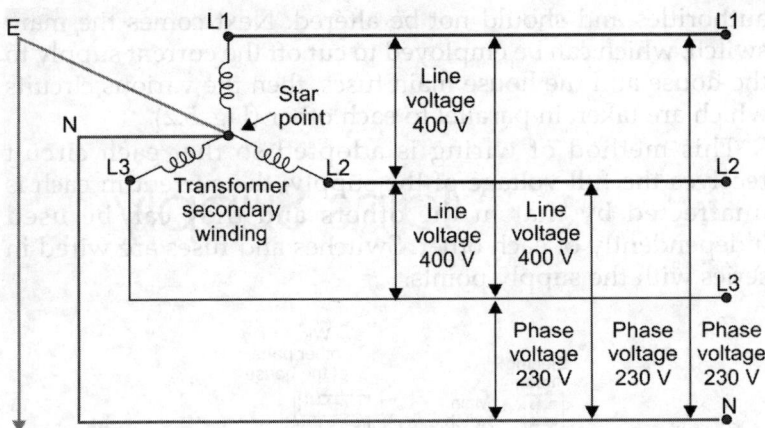

Fig. 5.1: Mains electricity supply (grid system), L1, L2, L3 are live wires, N is neutral wire

The current from the power stations is fed into a system of high-tension cables extending through the country. Where a district is to be supplied the cables are tapped and the voltage stepped down at a transformer station. One end of each of the secondary coils of the transformer is connected to earth and distribution throughout the local area is again by three live wires and one neutral wire. Each consumer receives one of the live wires and one neutral wire. As the current is alternating, the live wire is alternately negative and positive, the neutral wire being at zero potential throughout.

Advantages of grid system
1. All areas supplied by the system receive same voltage and type of current.
2. Large demands in one area do not put an excessive load on any particular power station.
3. Breakdown of one power station does not cut off the supply to any area.
4. Maintenance work is facilitated as all the generators are not necessary to be in operation all the time.

Wiring of the Houses (7 Marks)

The current on entering the house passes through the main fuses, and the meter, which are the property of the supply authorities and should not be altered. Next comes the main switch, which can be employed to cut off the current supply to the house and the house main fuses, then the various circuits which are taken in parallel to each other (Fig. 5.2).

This method of wiring is adopted so that each circuit receives the full voltage of the supply, the current in each is unaffected by that in the others and they can be used independently of each other. Switches and fuses are wired in series with the supply points.

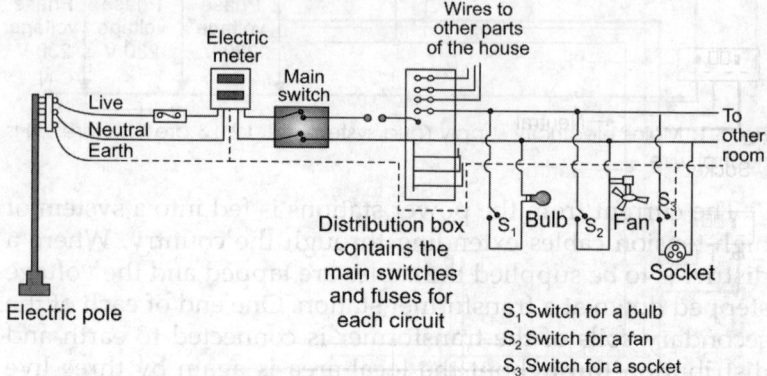

Fig. 5.2: Mains electricity distribution in a house

Light and Power Circuits

The circuits in the house can be divided into two categories: The light and the power circuits.

Light circuit: It has 5 ampere fuse for each 4–6 light circuit and the wiring to light circuit is design to carry slightly a larger intensity of current than a fuse.

Power circuit: It includes a fuse for each supply point. 13-ampere fuses are used in modern wiring and 15-ampere fuses in the wiring of older construction, and the cables can carry slightly larger intensity of current than the fuses.

The power circuits may be arranged in various ways:
1. A ring main: A complete loop is taken from each of the two supply cables and supply points are wired in parallel with each other between the loops. Fused plugs are used, so no fuses are incorporated in the wiring of individual

points, but a 30 ampere fuse is placed on the live wire entering the ring (Fig. 5.3).

The cable carries current from both sides of the loop, that is from two wires, each of which can carry at least 15 amperes; hence the high rating of the fuse. In large building there may be several rings, each with its own 30 ampere fuse.

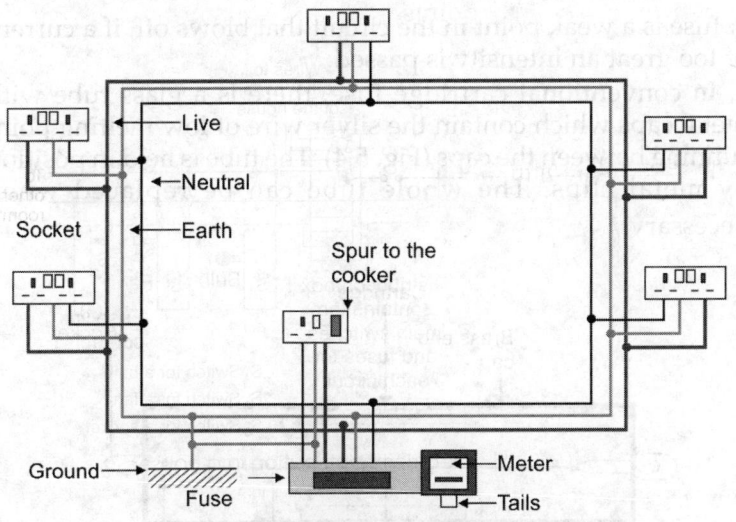

Fig. 5.3: The ring main

2. In addition to above, sub-circuits may be used for different installations such as an electric cooker or immersion heater or in the physiotherapy department, for certain equipment such as apparatus which uses a particularly large current.
3. In some cases light and power circuits divide immediately on entering the building and separate meters are provided, this method being used if different rates are charged for light and power.

The apparatus using a current of more than 5 amperes (A) must be connected to a power circuit or the intensity of current will exceed that which the fuse can transmit. Apparatus using a current of less than 5 A can be used on either type of circuit, but if the current is liable to approach 5 A, it is unwise to connect it to the light point. Moreover several light circuits are usually taken parallel to each other from one fuse and the current that passes through the fuse is the sum of that in the individual circuits. Consequently, the use of apparatus taking 4.5 A at one point would seriously limit the use of others.

Cartridge Fuse (3 Marks)

A fuse is a weak point in the circuit that blows off, if a current of too great an intensity is passed.

In conventional cartridge fuse, there is a glass tube with metal caps which contain the silver wire of low melting point running between the caps (Fig. 5.4). The tube is held in position by metal clips. The whole tube can be replaced when necessary.

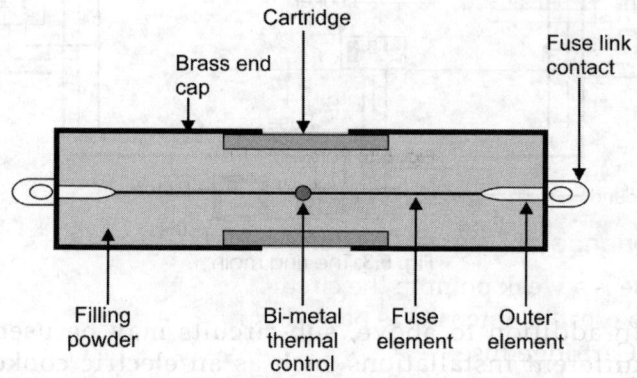

Fig. 5.4: Cartridge fuse

Porcelain Fuse (3 Marks)

The conventional porcelain fuse consists of a piece of suitable wire of low melting point running through the tunnel in a porcelain holder.

Each end of wire is attached by a screw to a metal blade. The blades fit into metal sockets in a fixed porcelain base and the main wire is connected to the sockets (Fig. 5.5).

The section containing the fuse wire can be removed for inspection and renewal of the wire.

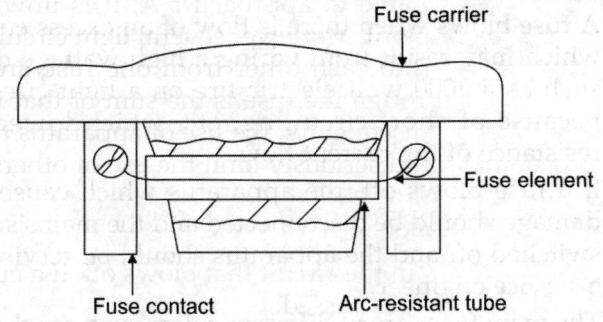

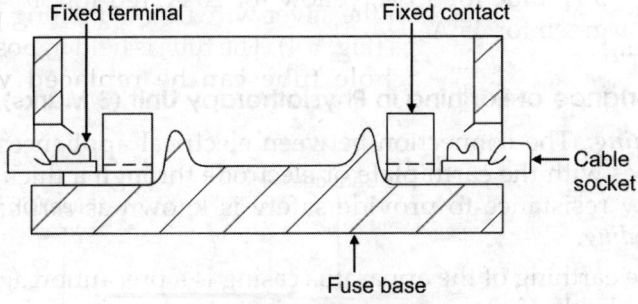

Fig. 5.5: Porcelain fuse

Importance of Fuses in Physiotherapy Unit (7 Marks)

A fuse is a weak point in the circuit that blows off, if a current of too great an intensity is passed. Fuses are of two types:

1. Cartridge fuse
2. Porcelain fuse.
   - It consists of a wire of low melting point so that when a large current passes, the wire melts breaking the circuit, stopping the flow of current.
   - The fuse should always break the live wire of the circuit if a single fuse is used and where two fuses are used it breaks both the live and the neutral wire.
   - The individual machines in the department should have their own fuses besides a fuse for the whole department.
   - The fuses should be placed at places which are easily accessible.

- A fuse blows when there is flow of an excess current, which may result from wiring a high wattage device such as a 2000 watt electric fire on a light circuit or because of short circuiting, etc. which lowers the resistance of the current flow.
- If a fuse blows off, the apparatus which caused the damage should be disconnected and the mains supply switched off and the apparatus should be serviced by a service engineer.
- The main fuses are of different colors such as white for 5 A, blue for 15 A, yellow for 20 A, red for 30 A and green for 45 A.

Importance of Earthing in Physiotherapy Unit (3 Marks)

Earthing: The connection between electrical appliances and devices with the earth plate or electrode through a thick wire of low resistance to provide safety is known as *earthing* or *grounding*.

The earthing of the apparatus casing is a precaution against earth shock. If the apparatus casing is not connected to the earth and the insulation on the live wire becomes worn so that this wire comes in contact with the casing.

Any connection between the casing and the earth completes a circuit through which current passes. If this connection is through a person he receives an earth shock. However, correct earthing of the casing has the effect that immediately the live wire comes in contact with it, current passes by the earth wire from the casing to earth.

This is a pathway of low resistance, so the current flow is great and the fuse on the live wire should blow. This stops the current flow and gives warning of the defect. Hence, earthing prevents excessive passage of current through the apparatus to the patient.

Power Plugs (3 Marks)

- All pieces of equipment working on a power circuit should be connected to the supply by a three-pin wall plug (Fig. 5.6). The pins that fit into the power sockets are

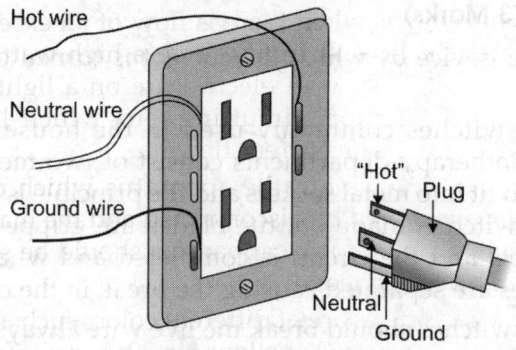

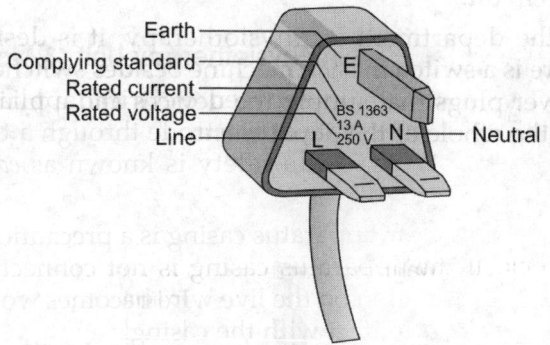

Fig. 5.6: Power plugs

arranged in a triangle, two being similar and the third (earth pin) being either large or differently spaced from others, so that the plug can be inserted into the socket in one way only.

- The two similar pins connect the apparatus with the supply and are marked 'L' and 'N' for the live and the neutral wires, respectively. The wires that connect the 'L' pin are either red or brown in color and that connect to the 'N' pin are either black or blue in color. The earth pin is connected to the wire with color of yellow or green which connect the outer casing of the apparatus to earth.
- Some plugs incorporate a fuse on the live wire which must not be capable of transmitting more than 13 A that the main wiring is designed to carry.

Switches (3 Marks)

Switch is a device by which the current is turned on and off (Fig. 5.7).

- The switches commonly used in the houses and the physiotherapy departments consist of two metal blades which fit into metal sockets and the principle is that when the switch is made on, the blades are gripped into the sockets and the circuit is completed and when off, the blades are separated causing the break in the circuit.

- The switches should break the live wire always but most satisfactory results are obtained if it breaks both wires of the circuit.

- In the department of physiotherapy, it is desired that there is a switch in each machine besides switches for the power plugs that supply the devices and a main switch for the whole of the department.

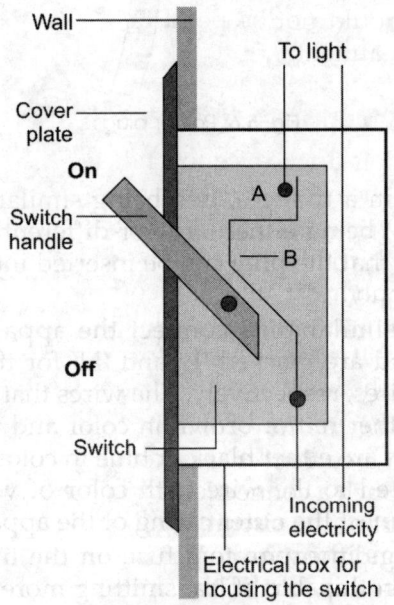

Fig. 5.7: Switches

SHOCK

Earth Shock (3 Marks)

When the shock is due to a connection between the live wire of the mains and the earth, it is known as earth shock.

The patient who is receiving treatment with a current that is not earth-free and if there is no earth connection between the outer casing of the apparatus and earth, there is every possibility that the person may form an earth circuit (provided that the floor is not insulated) through which the current is earthed resulting in earth shock. This can be made by touching any conductor which is connected to earth, e.g. gas or water pipes, metal bed on damp stone floor form an earth connection.

Precautions Against Earth Shock

a. The floor should be always of insulating material and it should be always dried.
b. Metal casing of all apparatus must be connected to earth.
c. Fuses must be on the live wire and switches must break the live wire.
d. Patient should not be permitted to touch the apparatus during treatment.

Earth Shock (7 Marks)

When the shock is due to a connection between the live wire of the mains and the earth, it is known as earth shock.

Electric power is transmitted by one live cable and one neutral cable which is connected to earth. The earth forms part of conducting pathway and any connection between the live wire of the main and earth completes a circuit through which current passes. If some person forms part of this circuit he receives an earth shock.

Connection to the live cable: A patient who is receiving treatment with a current that is not earth-free is connected to the live cable. Such a connection can also be made by touching an exposed part of the circuit, e.g. if the insulation on the live wire is faulty and the wire comes in contact with casing of the apparatus, then this part of the apparatus will also provide a connection to the live cable.

Connection to earth: This may be made by touching any conductor which is connected to earth, such as gas or water pipes or stone floors, particularly if they are damp. A metal bed on such a floor, or one which is in contact with a pipe, forms an earth connection.

Simultaneous connection to the live wire and to the earth can occur in the following ways:

a. A patient who is receiving treatment with a current that is not earth-free may rest his/her hand on water pipe or gas pipe.

b. A physiotherapist holding an electrode that is connected to live wire may come in contact with the earthed apparatus casing which may complete the circuit.

c. If someone standing on damp stone floor touches the casing of apparatus which is not connected to earth and with which the live wire is in contact, he will also receive an earth shock.

Precautions Against Earth Shock

1. Water and gas pipes should be out of reach of apparatus and patients receiving treatment.
2. The floor should be always of insulating material and it should be kept dry.
3. Metal casing of all apparatus must be connected to earth.
4. Special care must be taken when the current is given through bath. Water should not be added to the bath during treatment.
5. Fuses must be on the live wire and switches must break the live wire.
6. A current which is used for the treatment of the patient should always earth-free and to make the current earth-free use static transformer.
7. Patient should not be permitted to touch the apparatus during treatment.

Electric Shock (3 Marks)

It is a painful stimulation of sensory and motor nerves, caused by a sudden flow, cessation of flow or variation of intensity of current passing through the body, resulting in mild discomfort and fear to loss of consciousness and death in a few cases.

In physiotherapy department a shock can be caused by poorly designed or badly serviced electromedical apparatus, faulty handling of equipment and poor patient preparations.

Depending on the severity, shock can be classified: Mild shock or severe shock.

Following a mild shock: The victim may be frightened and may get a painful sensory stimulation. There may be breathing difficulty but no loss of consciousness.

Following a severe shock: The victim may remain connected to the circuit, there may be muscular paralysis; fall in blood pressure, ventricular fibrillation, loss of consciousness, cessation of respiration and cardiac arrest.

Electric Shock (7 Marks)

An electric shock is a painful stimulation of sensory and motor nerves, caused by a sudden flow, cessation of flow or variation of intensity of current passing through the body, resulting in mild discomfort and fear to loss of consciousness and death in a few cases.

In the department of physiotherapy a shock results from either due to poorly designed or badly serviced electro-medical apparatus, faulty operation of equipment and poor patient preparations.

The measure of the shock intensity is the amount of current passed through the body that causes the damage. The greater the current which passes through the body, the more severe is the shock. Shocks are generally more severe with alternating than with direct current.

Causes of electric shock: A person may obtain a shock without touching the active wire of the power supply by the following ways:

Sudden alteration of the current flow: If a low or medium frequency current is switched on with the controls turned up or if insufficient time is allowed for the apparatus to warm up, so that the current comes on suddenly after the controls have been turned up, it results in a sudden flow of current giving shock. Shock may also occur if the intensity control is turned up unduly during the intervals in the flow of an interrupted or surged current.

Improper earth connection: Many electrical apparatus have metal casings. An active voltage can be actually shortened to the casing because of the dropping of the instrument, moisture, deterioration of the equipment due to misuse or age. A person (patient/therapist) touching the casing could get a shock.

Leakage of currents: In all pieces of electrical equipment the intended current carrying parts are separated from the rest of the equipment by insulators. With high quality insulation and good circuit designs, there will be no problem with leakage currents but with poor designs, the leakage current from the wires carrying the current will be hazardous.

Two-pin connections: It is important that all electrical equipment should have a three-pin connection with the earth connection to avoid the leakage currents and hazards from metal casings. The three-pin system offers the protection of the fuse blowing, if there is a leakage or metal causing short circuit. The three-pin system has the protective ground connection, is the first to be plugged in and the last to be unplugged. The building itself must carry a good grounding system for the power supply. If the above features are absent and a two-pin connection is used it may give the shock.

Faulty electrical components: The presence of faulty components such as a faulty transformer or a leaky capacitor may be hazardous giving electric shock.

Non-insulated floorings: It is mandatory to have the floor of the electrotherapy unit to the insulated through vinyl or some other insulated floorings. If the floor is not insulated it enhances the occurrence of the earth shock.

Faulty switch and fuse connection: It is essential that the switches and fuses must break the live wire, if not it may produce shock.

Features of Electric Shock

Following a mild shock: The victim may be frightened and distressed, may get a painful sensory stimulation. There may be breathing difficulty but no loss of consciousness.

Following a severe shock: The victim may remain connected to the circuit, there may be muscular paralysis; fall in blood pressure, ventricular fibrillation, loss of consciousness, cessation of respiration and cardiac arrest.

The cessation of respiration is recognized by lack of respiratory movements and cyanosis, whereas the cardiac arrest can be recognized by the absence or abnormality of respiratory movements, absence of pulse in the carotid artery and fully dilated pupils.

Treatment of Electric Shock

- In the event of electric shock, the first step is to disconnect the victim from the contact with the current source. The current should be switched off at once.

- If there is no switch in the circuit the victim must be removed from contact with the conductor, but the rescuer must take care not to receive a shock himself by touching the affected person. The contact with the affected person should only be made by a thick layer of insulated material. After the person is removed a medical officer is immediately consulted and the following steps are taken.

- If the shock is a minor one, the victim is reassured and given rest. The victim may be given water to drink but hot drinks should be avoided as they cause vasodilatation and sweating and a further fall in blood pressure.

- If the shock is more severe, the victim is laid flat in such a position that the respiratory passages are clear. The tight clothing should be loosened and plenty of air is circulated to avoid undue warming, as it causes vasodilatation and increases sweating. The external heat increases the metabolism and so the demand for oxygen also increases which is hazardous.

- If the patient is unconscious nothing is given by mouth. If the respiration has ceased, clear the airways and start artificial respiration by mouth to mouth or mouth to nose methods and proceed for oxygen administration by a bag and mask. In the event of cardiac arrest, start external cardiac massage with mouth to mouth or mouth to nose breathing.

Precautions Against Electric Shock

1. Ensure that the current used is earth-free.
2. Ensure that the switches and fuses break the live wire.
3. Ensure that the apparatus casing is connected to earth.
4. Ensure that the power plug has three pins, one for live, other for neutral and the third for earth.
5. Ensure that the patient does not touch the apparatus during treatment.
6. The floor should be always of insulating material and it should be kept dry.
7. Water and gas pipes should be out of reach of apparatus and patients receiving treatment.
8. While applying the treatment in baths ensure that, the bath is made from insulating material and there should be no leakage of water, which may make an earth connection.

International Color Coding of Electrical Supply (3 Marks)

All pieces of equipment working on a power circuit should be connected to the supply by a three-pin wall plug. The pins that fit into the power sockets are arranged in a triangle, two being

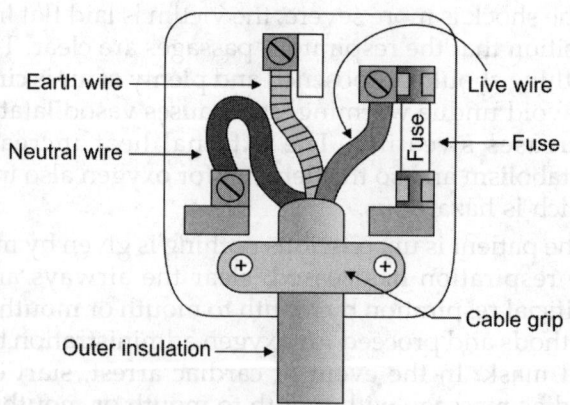

Fig. 5.8: Electrical plug with wiring

similar and the third (earth pin) being either large or differently spaced from others, so that the plug can be inserted into the socket in one way.

The two similar pins connect the apparatus with the supply and are marked L and N for the live and the neutral wires respectively. The wires that connect the L pin are either red or brown in color and that connect to the N pin are either black or blue in color. The earth pin is connected to the wire with color of green and yellow which connect the outer casing of the apparatus to earth (Fig. 5.8).

Basic Electrical Components

CAPACITOR (CONDENSER)

1. Basic Construction of a Capacitor (3 Marks)

The capacitor is a device for storing an electric charge, whose capacity can be changed without changing its shape and size.

In its simplest form it consists of two metal plates, which are separated by an insulated material called the dielectric (Fig. 6.1).

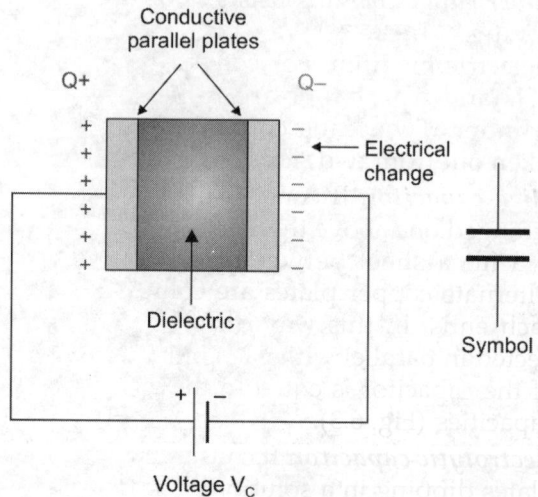

Fig. 6.1: Basic construction of a capacitor

When the plates are given opposite static electric charges, it leads to concentration of electric lines of force, leading to distortion of electron orbits of the atoms of the dielectric, thereby storing charges. The atoms of dielectric remain in this state of tension until the potential difference across the capacitor is removed.

When a condenser gets charged, there exists a difference of potential between its plates, which varies directly with the quantity of electricity with which it is charged, and inversely with the capacity of a condenser, i.e. $E = Q/C$

where E = Potential difference measured in volts.

Q = Quantity of electricity measured in Coulomb.

C = Capacity of condenser measured in farad.

2. Types of Capacitor (7 Marks)

All types of capacitor have the same basic construction: Two metal plates separated by an insulator (dielectric). The types are as follows:

1. **Fixed capacity capacitors:** These capacitors have fixed size of plates, fixed area and material of the dielectric, there by exhibiting fixed capacitance. The various types include:

   a. Paper capacitor: It consists of a pair of long tin foils having a piece of wax paper between them as a dielectric medium. For convenience purpose, the tin foils and wax paper are rolled into the form of a cylinder. Two leads connected to the two foils are taken out from two sides of the roll (Fig. 6.2).

   b. Mica capacitor: It consists of number of mica sheets arranged one above the other, in such a way that there is a mica sheet between every two copper plates. Alternate copper plates are connected to terminals at each ends. In this way different capacitors get connected in parallel with each other and the net capacity of the capacitor is equal to the sum of the individual capacities (Fig. 6.3).

   c. Electrolytic capacitor: It consists of a pair of aluminum plates dipping in a solution of aluminum borate. One plate is connected to the positive terminal and another

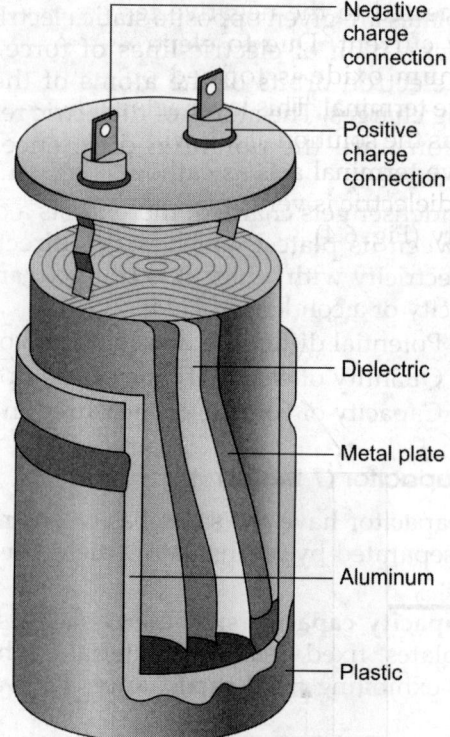

Fig. 6.2: Paper capacitor

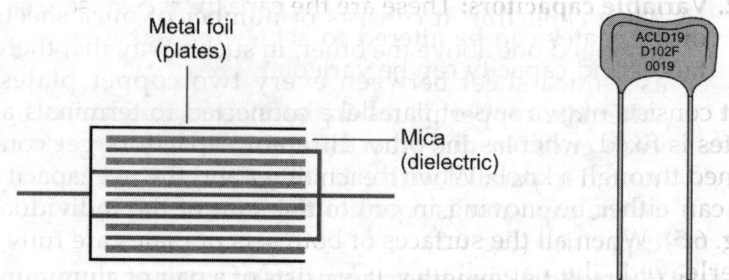

Fig. 6.3: Mica capacitor

is connected to the negative terminal of a source of steady current. Due to electrolysis a fine layer of aluminum oxide is formed on plate connected to positive terminal. This layer acts as dielectric medium, whereas the solution along with the plate connected to negative terminal acts as cathode. Since the thickness of the dielectric is very small, the capacitor has a large capacity (Fig. 6.4).

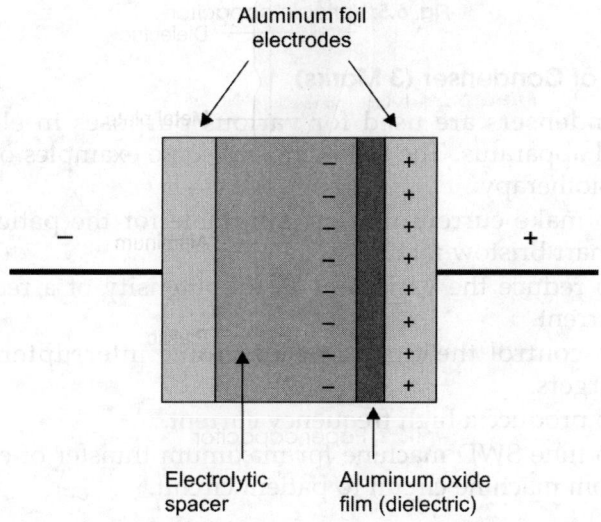

Aluminum foil electrodes

Electrolytic spacer

Aluminum oxide film (dielectric)

Fig. 6.4: Electrolytic capacitor

2. Variable capacitors: These are the capacitors, whose area of the plates can be altered to achieve variable capacitances and capacity can be varied at will.

It consists of two sets of parallel plates, in which one set of plates is fixed, whereas the other is capable of moving, when turned through a knob. When the knob is turned, the movable set can either be moving in or coming out of the fixed set (Fig. 6.5). When all the surfaces of both sets of plates are fully interleaved, the capacitance is at its maximum. Variable capacitors are found in short-wave diathermy machines, controlled by the 'tunning' knob.

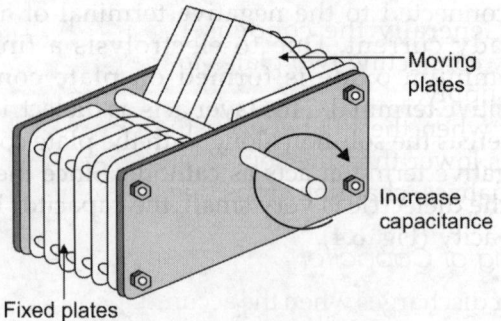

Fig. 6.5: Variable capacitor

3. Uses of Condenser (3 Marks)

The condensers are used for various purposes in electro-medical apparatus. The following are some examples of uses in physiotherapy:

1. To make current more comfortable for the patient, in Smart Bristow faradic coil.
2. To reduce the variations in the intensity of a rectified current.
3. To control the timing of electronic interrupters and surgers.
4. To produce a high frequency current.
5. To tune SWD machine for maximum transfer of energy from machine circuit to patient circuit.

4. Charging and Discharging of Capacitor
Or
Capacitor Discharge Through Low Ohmic Resistance (7 Marks)

Charging of Capacitor

A capacitor can be charged by electrostatic induction, where a static electric charge is allowed to build up on the plates of the capacitor or directly by applying a potential difference across the plates from either the mains or battery.

To charge by electrostatic induction, one plate of the condenser is connected to a source of supply, so that it acquires a positive or negative charge and the other plate is connected to earth. Generally the condenser is made to be charged directly, by connecting two plates to the opposite poles of the source of supply.

Initially when the PD between the plates of the charging capacitor is lower than the source, charging is greater, but as the PD equalizes, charging stops (Fig. 6.6a).

Discharging of Capacitor

A capacitor discharges when the accumulated charge is allowed to flow off the plates. If the two plates with opposite charges are connected, electrons flow from the negative to the positive plate until their charges are equal. The time taken for this discharge depends on the capacitance of the condenser, the resistance of the pathway and the quantity of the electricity involved.

Initially as the PD between the plates of a charged condenser is greater than the circuit through which the condenser is made to discharge, the discharging is fast, but as the PD between the two equalizes the discharging stops (Fig. 6.6b).

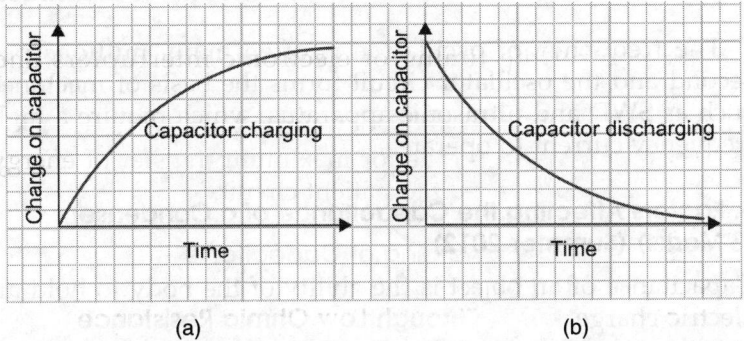

(a)   (b)

Fig. 6.6a and b: Graph showing charging and discharging of capacitor

Capacitor Discharge Through Low Ohmic Resistance or Oscillator Circuit

If the charged capacitor is discharged through a circuit of low ohmic resistance which includes an inductance (a coil of wire), electrons flow forward then back between the plates in an oscillating manner. The reason for this sequence of events is that as current flows through the inductance, self-induced

EMFs are produced. These back EMFs impede electron flow, but when both plates reach the same potential, the forward EMF causes an electron flow onto one plate with the result that it becomes negatively charged. This sequence continues as a series of damped oscillations until all the energy in the system is exhausted (Fig. 6.7).

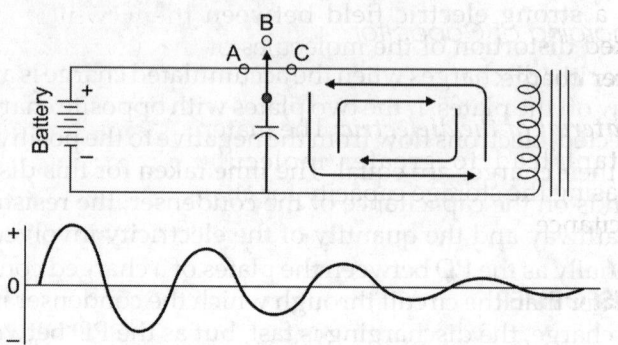

Fig. 6.7: Damped oscillation caused by resistance in the circuit

The frequency of oscillation is often many millions per second and the oscillator circuit forms the basis of machines such as SWD and ultrasonic apparatus, which require a high frequency current to operate.

5. Factors Affecting the Capacitance of a Condenser (3 Marks) (Summer 2012)

Capacitance of an object is the ability of the body to hold an electric charge.

It is measured in *farads*, although for practical purposes the *microfarad* (10^{-6} farad) is used.

Capacitance of a condenser depends upon the following factors:

Area of plates: The capacitance of a condenser depends on the area of the plates. When area of condenser increases its potential decreases; therefore, capacity of condenser increases with area.

Material of the plates: As some materials are good conductors than others, the condenser with plates made from a good conductor has large capacity, than the one made from plates of low conducting material.

Width of the dielectric: If the condenser has a dielectric medium that is thin, there is a strong force of attraction between the opposite charges on each side of it. This leads to concentration of charges on the adjacent surfaces of the plates, with a strong electric field between them, which leads to marked distortion of the molecules of the dielectric, storing a greater charge.

Material of the dielectric: The materials with high dielectric constant lead to greater molecular distortion, thereby increasing the storage capacity for charges and hence a greater capacitance.

TRANSFORMER

Types of Transformers (7 Marks)

Transformer is a device used for changing low alternating voltage at high current. It changes the alternating voltage without the loss of energy.

The transformers are divided into three types: Static transformer, variable transformer and autotransformer.

Static transformer: The static transformer (Fig. 6.8) is based on the principle of electromagnetic induction and is used to alter voltage of an alternating current and to render the current earth-free.

Construction: It consists of 2 coils, primary and secondary coils, which are completely insulated from each other and wound on a laminated soft iron frame. The frame is often rectangular in shape and the coils may be wound on opposite bars of the frame or one on top of the other on a central bar.

Working of the static transformer: An alternating current is passed through the primary coil that sets up a varying magnetic field, which cuts the secondary coil and induces an EMF in it. There is no electrical connection between primary and secondary coils, the energy being transmitted from one to

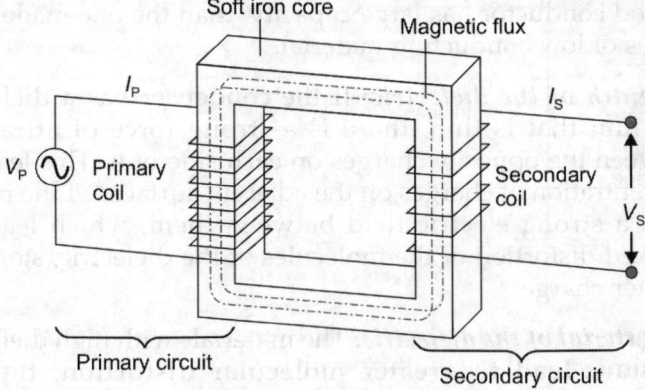

Fig. 6.8: Static transformer

the other by electromagnetic induction. The core serves to concentrate the magnetic field and it is laminated to prevent eddy currents.

Types of Static Transformer

1. *Step-up transformer:* If the number of turns in the secondary coil is more than that of the primary, the voltage-induced in the secondary coil will be increased or stepped up. Such a device is called step-up transformer (Fig. 6.9).
2. *Step-down transformer:* If the number of turns in the secondary coil is less than that of the primary, the voltage induced in the secondary coil will be decreased or stepped down. Such a device is called step-down transformer (Fig. 6.10).

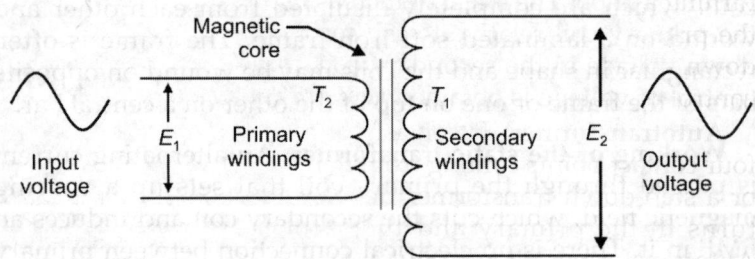

Fig. 6.9: Step-up transformer

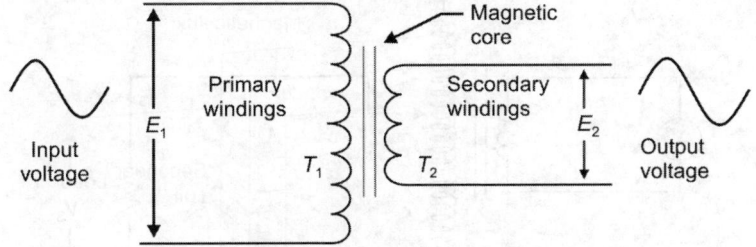

Fig. 6.10: Step-down transformer

3. *Even-ratio transformer:* If the number of turns in the primary and secondary coil is same, the voltage in the primary is same as that of the secondary. Such a device is called even-ratio transformer (Fig. 6.11).

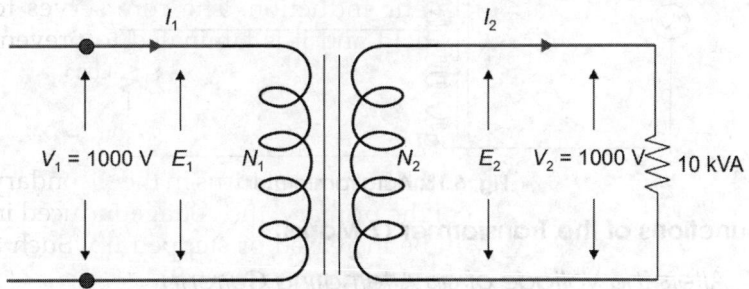

Fig. 6.11: Even-ratio transformer

Variable transformer: It consists of primary and secondary coils, but is constructed so that one of them can be altered in length. The primary coil has a number of tapings taken from it and a movable contact can be made on any one of these by turning a knob. The effect of increasing the number of turns in the primary coil relative to the secondary is to cause a step-down voltage in the secondary coil. In this way a very crude control of voltage is obtained (Fig. 6.12).

Autotransformer: It consists of a single coil of wire with four contact points coming from it. It can be used as a step-up, or a step-down transformer depending upon the number of turns in the primary and the secondary coils (Fig. 6.13). Autotransformer allows only a small step-up of voltage and does not render the current earth-free.

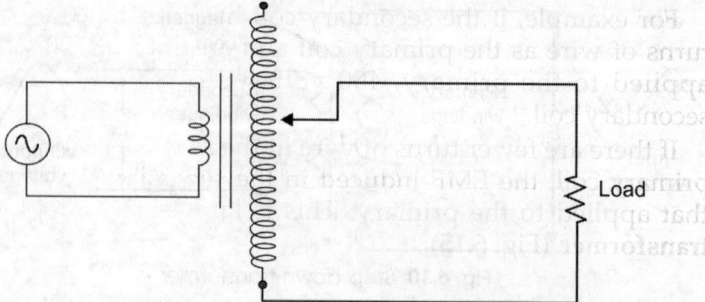

Fig. 6.12: Variable transformer

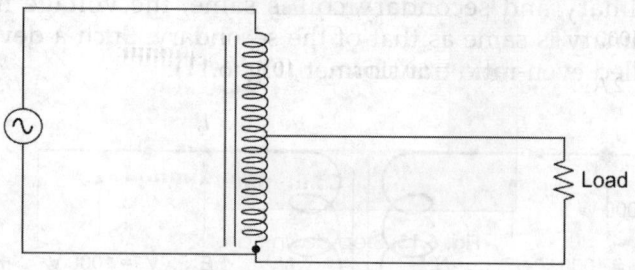

Fig. 6.13: Autotransformer

Functions of the Transformer (7 Marks)

1. Alters the Voltage of an Alternating Current

The EMF-induced in the secondary coil depends upon the number of turns of wire it has, relative to the primary coil.

If there are more turns of wire in the secondary than in the primary coil, the EMF obtained from the secondary is greater than that applied to the primary. This is known as a **step-up transformer** (Fig. 6.14).

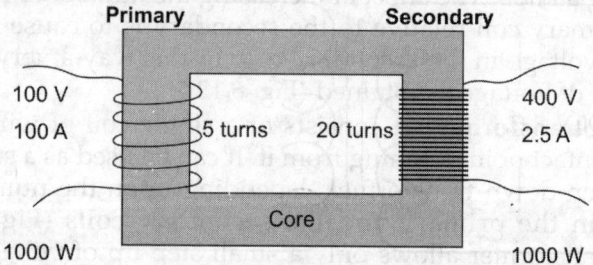

Fig. 6.14: Step-up transformer

For example, if the secondary coil has four times as many turns of wire as the primary coil and an EMF of 100 volts is applied to the primary, 400 volts will be induced in the secondary coil.

If there are fewer turns of wire in the secondary than in the primary coil, the EMF induced in the secondary is less than that applied to the primary. This is known as a **step-down transformer** (Fig. 6.15).

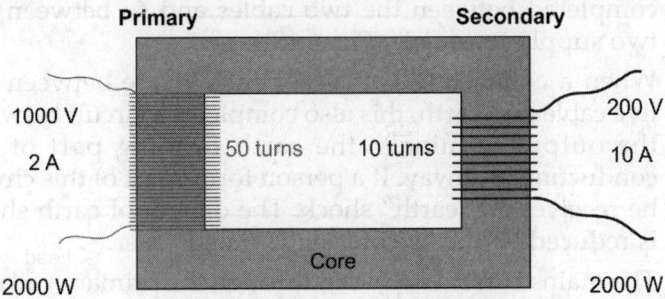

Fig. 6.15: Step-down transformer

For example, if the primary coil has five times as many turns of wire as the secondary coil and an EMF of 1000 volts is applied to the primary, 200 volts will be induced in the secondary coil.

If there are the same number of turns of wire in both coils the EMF induced in the secondary is the same as that applied to the primary. This is known as an **even-ratio transformer** (Fig. 6.16). Its sole function is to render the current earth-free.

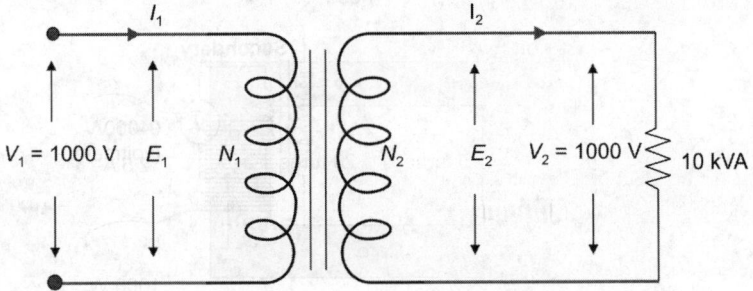

Fig. 6.16: Even-ratio transformer

2. Renders a Current Earth-free

The consumer is supplied by two cables, the live and neutral wires. The live wire is insulated from earth and is electrically charged. The neutral wire is connected to earth at intervals along its course and it is always at zero potential.

- Most electrical apparatus works on a current, which flows from the live wire, through the apparatus, to the neutral wire and earth. When a current is required, a circuit is completed between the two cables and so between the two supply terminals (Fig. 6.17).

- When a connection is inadvertently made between the live cable and earth, this also completes a circuit between the output terminals, the earth forming part of the conducting pathway. If a person forms part of this circuit he receives an "earth" shock. The danger of earth shock is reduced by the use of a static transformer.

- The mains current is passed through the primary coil and induces an EMF in the secondary coil. There is no electrical connection between the primary and secondary coils; the latter has no connection to earth. The earth does not form any part of the conducting pathway of the secondary current, which is said to be earth-free.

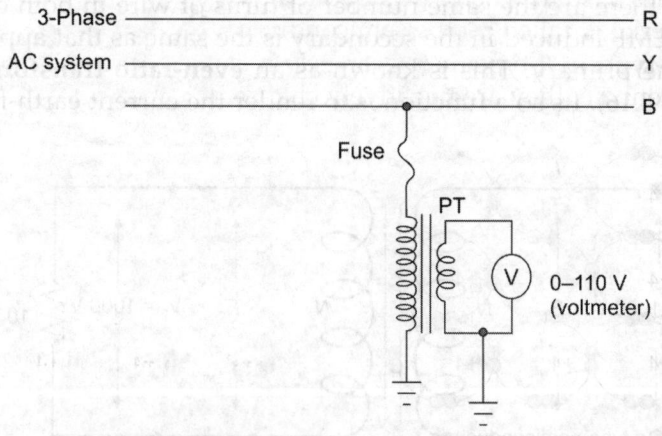

Fig. 6.17: An earthed circuit

- The transformer renders the current earth-free as long as there is no electrical connection between primary and secondary coils. If the insulation between the coils break down the secondary circuit would be connected to earth and there would be danger of earth shock.

SEMICONDUCTOR

1. Semiconductor and its Types (7 Marks)

Semiconductors are usually metal which because of thermal agitation or the addition of impurities have electrons free to conduct current.

Semiconductors are classified into *p*-type and *n*-type (Fig. 6.18).

p-type: In *p*-type there is deficiency of electron which gives rise to positive 'holes', due to which current flow occurs, i.e. they are positively charged materials.

When certain materials such as aluminum with atomic no. 13 (3 electrons in outer shell) are added to an atom of silicon with atomic no. 14 (4 electrons in outer shell) then three outer electrons of aluminum make covalent bond with three electrons in the outer orbit of silicon, whereas for the 4th there is no electron available on the outer orbit of aluminum, creating an electron deficiency called positive hole which carries current when PD is applied to such a material. Such a material is called *p*-type semiconductors.

n-type: In *n*-type there is an excess of electron which carries current, i.e. they are negatively charged materials.

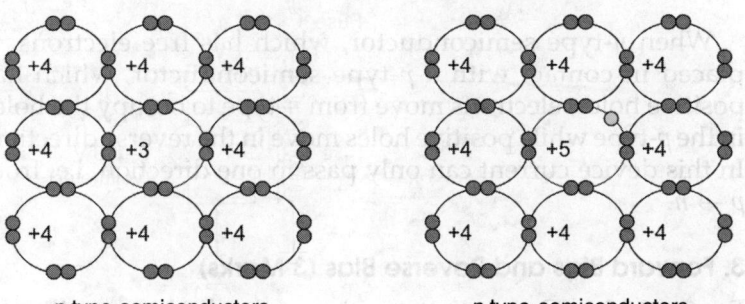

p-type semiconductors   n-type semiconductors

Fig. 6.18: Types of semiconductors

When certain materials such as phosphorus with atomic no. 15 (5 electrons in outer shell) are added to an atom of silicon with atomic no. 14 (4 electrons in outer shell) then four electrons of phosphorus make covalent bond with four electrons of silicon, leaving behind one free electron in the phosphorus which carries current when PD is applied to such a material. Such a material is called *n*-type semiconductors.

If a *p*- and an n-type of semiconductor are fused together, current can only pass in the $n \rightarrow p$ direction and the semiconductor therefore act as a valve.

2. Semiconductor Diode (3 Marks)

An electronic device created by bringing together a *p*-type and *n*-type region within the same semiconductor lattice is called semiconductor diode (Fig. 6.19).

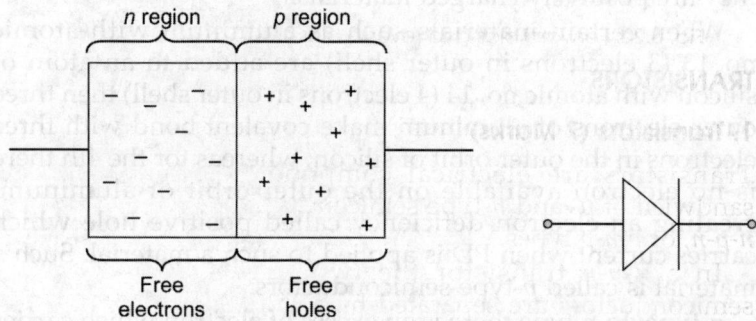

Fig. 6.19: Semiconductor diode and its symbol

When *n*-type semiconductor, which has free electrons, is placed in contact with a *p*-type semiconductor, which has positive holes, electrons move from *n*-type to occupy the holes in the *p*-type while positive holes move in the reverse direction. In this device current can only pass in one direction, i.e. from $p \rightarrow n$.

3. Forward Bias and Reverse Bias (3 Marks)

Forward bias: Connecting positive of the diode to positive of the supply and negative of the diode to negative of the supply.

It is the condition that permits current through the *p-n* junction of a diode (Fig. 6.20a).

Reverse bias: Connecting positive of the diode to negative of the supply and negative of diode to positive of the supply (Fig. 6.20b). In this condition the *depletion region* widens until its potential difference equals the bias voltage, majority-carrier current ceases.

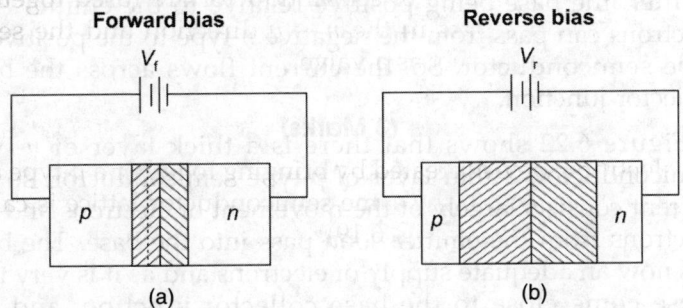

Fig. 6.20: Forward bias and reverse bias at semiconductor diode

TRANSISTORS

1. Transistors (7 Marks)

Transistors are electrical components, which utilize a sandwich of *p*- and *n*-type semiconductor materials. It can be *n-p-n*, or *p-n-p* types.

In a *n-p-n* transistor the two thick layers of *n*-type semiconductors are separated by a thin layer of *p*-type. The part where electrons enter the transistor is called the *emitter*, the central part the *base*, and the part where electrons leave, the *collector*. One of the *n*-type at the left is the emitter, the other at the right is the collector, and the central *p*-type is the base (Fig. 6.21).

On contact being made between materials, say *n-p-n* semiconductors in this case, PD develops at their junctions,

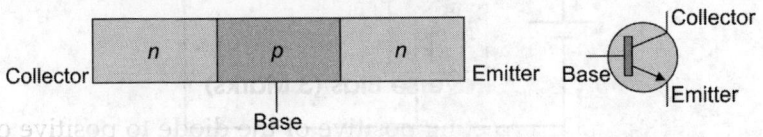

Fig. 6.21: *n-p-n* transistor

the emitter and the collector, being positive relative to the base. When the device is connected to a source of EMF, with the emitter negative and the collector positive, no current flows unless the EMF exceeds the critical value, as the electrons are unable to the pass from the negative *p*-type to the positive *n*-type semiconductor, so cannot cross the base collector junction.

A second source of EMF is connected to the base and the emitter, the base being positive relative to the emitter. The electrons can pass from the negative *n*-type to the positive *p*-type semiconductor. So, the current flows across the base collector junction.

Figure 6.22 shows that there is a thick layer of *n*-type semiconductor, a thin layer of *p*-type semiconductor, so the current consists largely of the movement of electrons and the electrons from the emitter soon pass into the base. The base has now an adequate supply of electrons and as it is very thin these come close to the base collector junction, and are attracted into the collector to replace those that had migrated into the base. This reduces the barrier effect across the base-collector junction, and current flows across the transistor.

Thus, a current fed into the base renders the transistor capable of conducting current and small variations in this base current, causes greater variation of current flowing across the transistor.

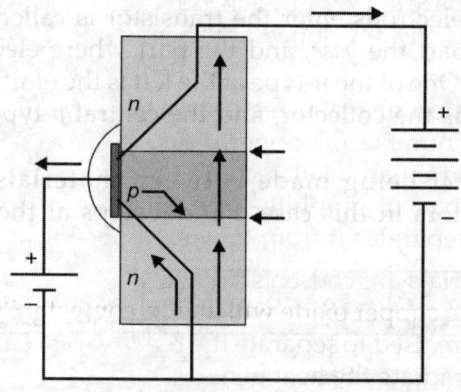

Fig. 6.22: *n-p-n* transistor

2. Uses of Transistor (3 Marks)

Uses of transistors are as follows:

1. Transistors are used in preference to the valves, in most modern electrical equipment, as they are durable, have a long life, consume less power and need no heating device.

2. As the power output is limited they are suitable for use in the production of low frequency but fail to produce high frequency currents, e.g. SWD.

METAL RECTIFIER

1. Metal Rectifier (7 Marks)

A metal rectifier works on the principles of semiconductor diode. One type of rectifier consists of a copper disc, coated on the surface with copper oxide. Copper oxide is a p-type of semiconductor and copper being a metal has free electrons, so acts like an n-type semiconductor. So, when the two materials are in contact, a PD develops at their junction.

When the rectifier is connected into a circuit with the copper negative (n-type) relative to the copper oxide (p-type), current passes more easily.

If the polarity is reversed, no current flows until the EMF exceeds certain level (8 volts).

A series of discs can be used to rectify larger voltages but must be separated from each other by suitable materials; otherwise the PD developed at the contacts would cancel each other out.

Construction of metal rectifier: The rectifier consists of an appropriate number of copper discs, oxidized on one surface and mounted on an insulated rod. In contact with the copper oxide is a layer of graphite, then a lead disc and aluminum cooling fin separates it from the next unit (Fig. 6.23).

The materials are chosen so that a PD develops only at that surface of the copper oxide which is in contact with the copper. Lead discs are used to separate the rectifying units. The cooling fin serve to radiate the heat generated which would otherwise interfere with the working.

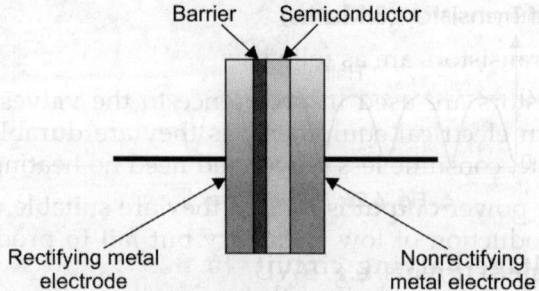

Fig. 6.23: Metal rectifier

2. Rectification of Alternating Current (AC) (7 Marks)

Rectification of an AC: Rectification is a process of conversion of alternating current (AC) into direct current (DC).

Types of rectification are

Half wave rectification: If one diode valve or metal rectifier is included in the circuit, current can pass in one direction only and the flow is blocked during alternate half cycles of alternating current. The resulting current that is obtained is unidirectional, pulsating and interrupted, and the process by which it is obtained is called half wave rectification (Fig. 6.24).

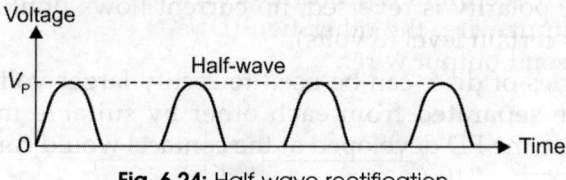

Fig. 6.24: Half-wave rectification

Full-wave rectification: It is the process by which a unidirectional, pulsating but uninterrupted current flow is produced. The circuits that produce the full-wave rectification are such that, the direction of the current is reversed during alternate half cycles of AC (Fig. 6.25).

Examples of circuits which produce full-wave rectification are:

1. Voltage-halving circuit
2. The Westinghouse Bridge

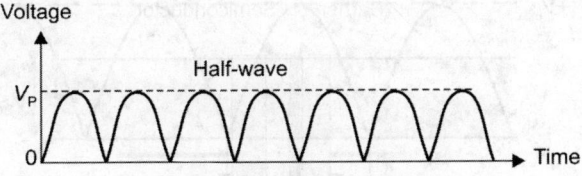

Fig. 6.25: Full-wave rectification

1. **Voltage-halving circuit**: In this circuit, two metal rectifiers or a diode with two anodes are connected to each end of secondary coil of the transformer. The center of the secondary coil is connected to the other lead.

Figure 6.26 shows when A is negative and B is positive, current cannot flow round the circuit from A as it is unable to cross the valve in this direction. It therefore passes from C round the external circuit and back to B. When A is positive and B is negative, current flows from C, through the external circuit and back to A. The resultant output waveform is shown in Fig. 6.27.

2. **The Westinghouse Bridge**: In this four blocks of rectifiers are used in a diamond arrangement, the input wires being connected to the opposite corners of the diamond, and the output wires taken from the other two corners. Two rectifiers (D_1 and D_3) are directed towards one output wire, the other two (D_2 and D_4) away from the second output wire.

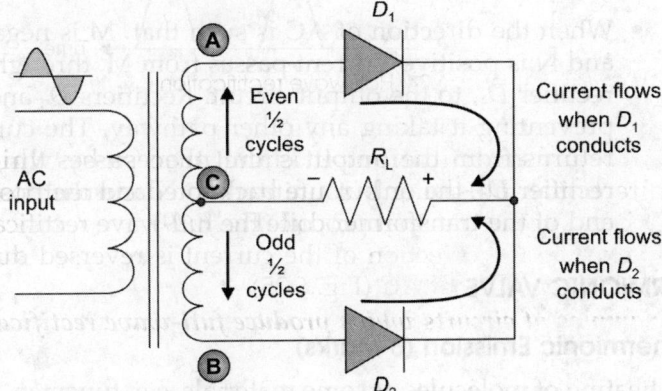

Fig. 6.26: Voltage-halving circuit

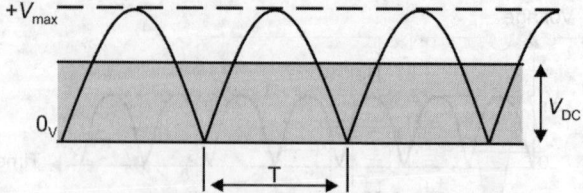

Fig. 6.27: Resultant output waveform

- When M is positive and N is negative, current passes from N through rectifier D_4, round the output circuit and back by rectifier D_3 to M. Thus, the current always passes in the same direction through the output circuit, and full-wave rectification is obtained (Fig. 6.28). There is some drop in voltage, owing to the resistance of the rectifiers, but it is very less than that which occurs in voltage-halving circuit.

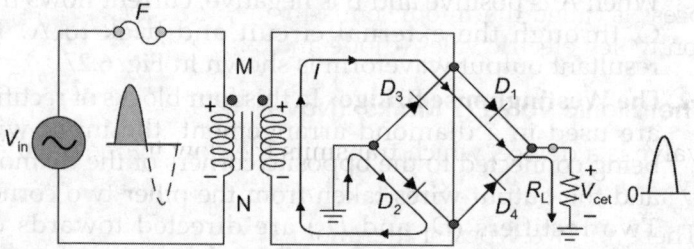

Fig. 6.28: During positive half cycle of input—D1 and D2 are forward biased and conduct current

- When the direction of AC is such that, M is negative and N is positive, current passes from M, through the rectifier D_1, to the output circuit. Rectifiers D_3 and D_4 preventing it taking any other pathway. The current returns from the output circuit then passes through rectifier D_2, the only route back to N and the positive end of the transformer coil (Fig. 6.29).

THERMIONIC VALVE

1. Thermionic Emission (3 Marks)

The heating of molecules of some materials, e.g. tungsten, may cause molecular agitation that some electrons leave their atoms

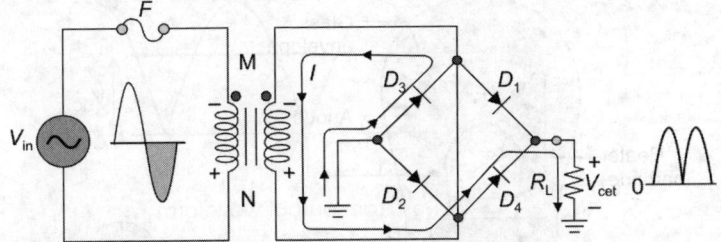

Fig. 6.29: During negative half cycle of input—D_3 and D_4 are forward biased and conduct current

and may even break free of the surface of the metal. This leaves a positive charge on the atom which tends to attract the negative electrons back. However, a point is reached where the rate of loss of electrons exceeds the rate of return and a cloud of electrons then exists as a space charge around the object. The process is called thermionic emission and this is the principle upon which electric vales (diode and triode) work.

2. Thermionic Valve (7 Marks) (Nov-Dec 2010)

A valve is a device, which transmits the flow in one direction only.

There are two types of thermionic valves:

1. Diode valve
2. Triode valve

Diode Valve

A diode valve consists of an evaluated glass tube into which are sealed two separate electrodes, i.e. cathode (filament) and anode (plate) (Fig. 6.30).

The filament used can be directly or indirectly heating type. The anode plate is made up of metal, which does not allow thermionic emission readily and it is in the form of a cylinder surrounding the cathode. For the current to pass through the valve, the filament must be heated, causing emission of electrons by the process of thermionic emission. The electrons so emitted will be attracted by the positive anode constituting an electrical current, when a PD is applied across the valve.

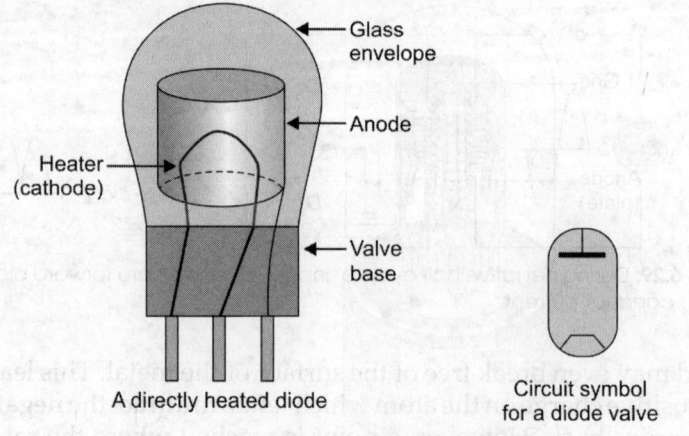

A directly heated diode

Circuit symbol for a diode valve

Fig. 6.30: Diode valve

When the applied PD is reversed, so that the plate (anode) is negative with respect to the cathode, no current flows through the valve, indicating that electrons can pass only from cathode to anode and not in the reverse direction.

Triode Valve

The triode valve is a device that contains three electrodes, viz. cathode, anode and the grid. The grid, whose potential can be altered, is placed between the cathode and anode (Fig. 6.31).

The triode valve works on exactly the same principle as the diode valve. When the filament will be heated as like the diode, current passes from the valve in one direction only. The grids, whose potential can be altered, have effect on current flow across the valve.

It is possible using an external circuit to make the grid – ve, + ve, or neutral.

If neutral the grid will not affect electron flow across the valve. If positive, it will attract electron away from the cathode and thus amplify the electron flow through the valve. If negative, the grid will repel electron and reduce or even stop the electron flow.

The charges applied to the grid from the external source are called *grid bias*. The flow of current across the triode valve can be regulated by adjusting the bias of the grid.

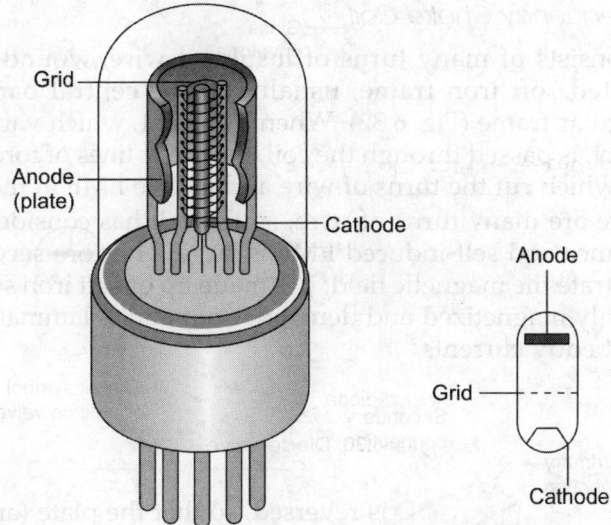

Fig. 6.31: Triode valve

3. Uses of Triode Valve (3 Marks)

1. Used for the production of high frequency currents in conjunction with a condenser and inductance.
2. Used for the production of interrupted current and other muscle stimulating currents.
3. It is not used as a rectifier, but rectifies the current that passes through it.
4. It is used as a switch.

CHOKE COIL

1. Choke Coil (7 Marks) (Summer 2012)

It is a device including in the circuit to produce self-induced EMF, maintaining a smooth flow of current.

Types of choke coil:
1. Low frequency choke coil
2. High frequency choke coil

Low Frequency Choke Coil

This consists of many turns of insulated wire, wound on a laminated soft iron frame, usually on the central bar of a rectangular frame (Fig. 6.32). When a current, which varies in intensity, is passed through the coil, magnetic lines of force are set up which cut the turns of wire and induce EMF in them.

There are many turns of wire, so the coil has considerable inductance and self-induced EMF is large. The core serves to concentrate the magnetic field; it is made up of soft iron so that it is easily magnetized and demagnetized and is laminated to prevent eddy currents.

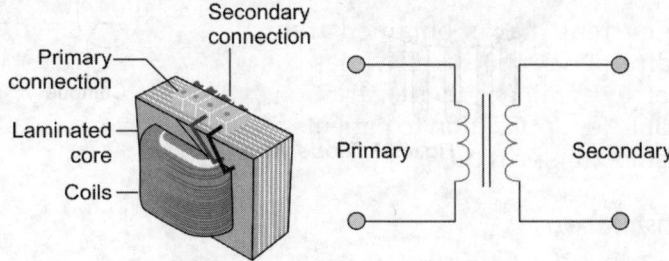

Fig. 6.32: Low frequency choke coil

High Frequency Choke Coil

This consists of several turns of insulated wire wound on a bobbin of some non-conducting material.

A high frequency current varies very rapidly in intensity so tends to produce a considerable self-induced EMF. Consequently, it is unnecessary to have many turns of wire in a high frequency choke coil, or to wind them on a soft iron core.

2. Uses of Choke Coil (3 Marks)

1. **To even out the variations in the intensity of the current, providing a smooth current flow:** The self-induced EMF which is set up when a varying current is passed through a choke coil retards the rise of current to maximum and prolongs the current flow, when the intensity is falling, thereby maintaining an even flow of current.

2. **To prevent the flow of a high frequency current and allow the passage of the low frequency one:** When a high frequency current is passed through a choke coil, the inductive reactance (the impedance to the flow of self-induced current) is considerable, thereby retarding the flow of such a current, whereas when a low frequency current is passed, the impedance to current flow considerably less than to a high frequency current, due to which the choke coil serves the above function.

SMOOTHING CIRCUIT

1. Smoothing Circuit (7 Marks)

The current that is obtained from the rectifying circuit is unidirectional, but it still varies considerably in intensity. In order to eliminate these variations and render the current suitable for application to patients, a circuit is necessary called the smoothing circuit.

Construction

The circuit consists of one or two condensers wired in parallel to the output circuit, and a choke coil in series with the circuit (Fig. 6.33).

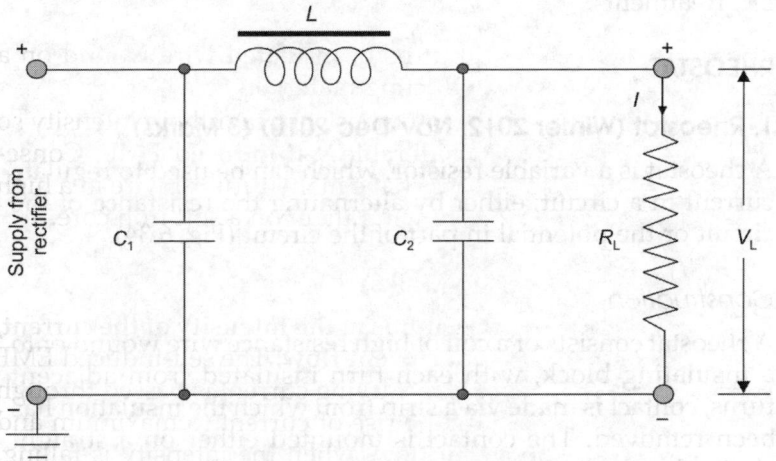

Fig. 6.33: Smoothing circuit

Working

When the EMS of the rectified current rises, current flows in the external circuit and at the same time the condensers are charged.

When the EMS falls, the intensity of the current in the output circuit falls but the condensers discharge round this circuit and augment the current flow so that the intensity does not fall to zero.

Thus, the variations in the intensity of the current are reduced. The condensers have a large capacity, so that they offer a little impedance to the charging current and hold a considerable quantity of electricity to discharge round the circuit.

As the current varies in intensity, a self-induced EMF is set up in the choke coil. When the intensity of the current is rising, the self-induced EMF opposes the applied EMF and retards the rising current.

When the intensity of the current is falling, the self-induced EMF is in the same direction as the applied EMF and prolongs the current flow. These effects further reduce the variations of the intensity of the currents.

The current that is obtained from the smoothing circuit varies slightly in intensity but it is still suitable for constant DC treatments.

RHEOSTAT

1. Rheostat (Winter 2012, Nov-Dec 2010) (3 Marks)

A rheostat is a variable resistor, which can be used to regulate current in a circuit; either by alternating the resistance of the circuit or the potential in part of the circuit (Fig. 6.34).

Construction

A rheostat consists of a coil of high resistance wire wound onto a insulating block, with each turn insulated from adjacent turns, contact is made via a strip from which the insulation has been removed. The contact is mounted either on a straight sliding bar or on a pivot turned by a knob.

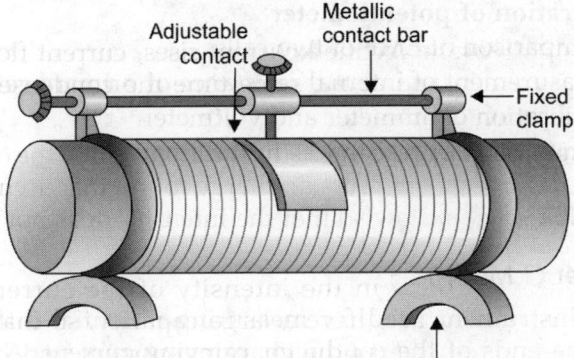

Fig. 6.34: Rheostat

Type of rheostat

1. Rotary rheostat

2. Shunt rheostat

3. Slide/linear rheostat

POTENTIOMETER

Potentiometer or Shunt Resistance (3 Marks)

State the Construction of Shunt Rheostat (Summer 2012)

Potentiometer is used to measure the EMF of any cell or potential difference between any two points in the circuit.

Construction

The base of the apparatus is a large wooden plank on which a very long wire (6–10 m) is fixed in such a way that, each one meter length is parallel to some of the other lengths of the same wire. A piece of 1 meter long wires are taken and connected in series by using thick brass stops at the junctions of the two wires. In this way the total length is made long.

The two ends of the wire are connected to screws M and N. Jockey (J) can be shifted to the plank and can be connected with any part of the wire.

Application of potentiometer

1. Comparison of EMF of two cells.
2. Measurement of internal resistance of primary cell.
3. Calibration of ammeter and voltmeter.
4. Comparison of resistances in the circuit.

VOLTMETER

Voltmeter (7 Marks)

It is an instrument used for measuring potential difference across the ends of the conductor carrying current. A galvanometer can be converted into voltmeter by connecting a high resistance in series with it.

Construction

A voltmeter is a pivoted coil type galvanometer (G), wired in series with high resistance (R). The coils attached with a light aluminum pointer, which can rotate in a circular scale having equispaced marks indicating volts (V) (Fig. 6.35).

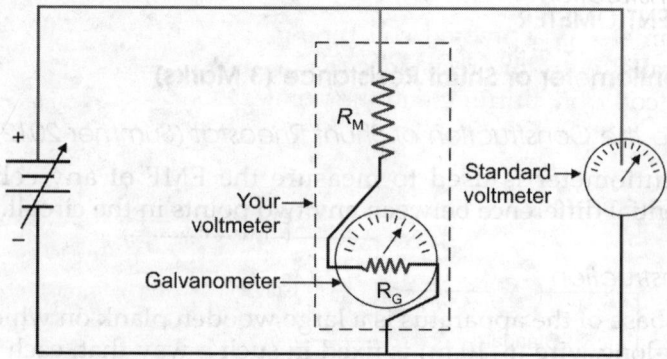

Fig. 6.35: Conversion of a galvanometer to a voltmeter

Wiring into the circuit

- The voltmeter is connected in **parallel** to the circuit, across which the potential difference (PD) is to be measured.

- A high resistance is connected in **series** to the coil of the galvanometer, so a very negligible amount of current is passed to the coil and thus the main current remains the same.

Features of a voltmeter

1. It is used to measure PD, between two points of an electrical circuit.
2. It is always connected in parallel with an electrical circuit.
3. A high resistance is connected in series with its coil. An ideal voltmeter has infinite resistance.

AMMETER

Ammeter (7 Marks)

It is an instrument used to measure current in an electrical circuit. The galvanometer can be converted into an ammeter by connecting a low resistance parallel to the galvanometer (Fig. 6.36). This low resistance (R) is called shunt resistance (S). This shunted galvanometer is called ammeter.

Construction

Ammeter is a pivoted coil type galvanometer (G), wired in parallel with low resistance (R) or shunt. The shunt protects the coil from burning and the pointer from breaking.

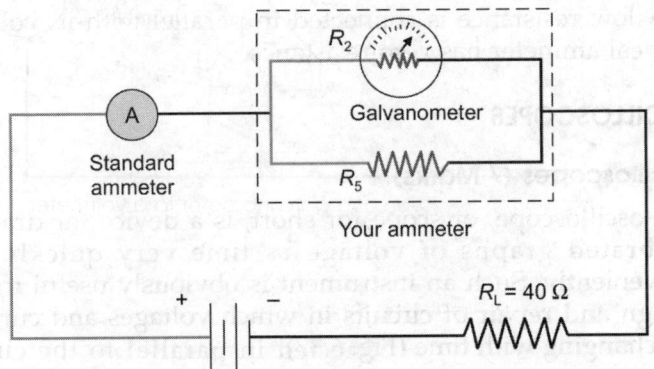

Fig. 6.36: Conversion of a galvanometer to an ammeter

The coil is attached with a light aluminum pointer which can rotate in a circular scale having equispaced marks indicating ampere (A).

Wiring into the Circuit

• The ammeter is always connected in series with the circuit. A low resistance is connected in parallel to the coil of the galvanometer, so that the resultant resistance becomes very low and almost all the current passes through the coil of the galvanometer.

• The current is always passed through (+) terminal to (–) terminal, as the pointer deflects from left to right only. Hence, its positive terminal should always be connected to positive terminal to prevent breaking of pointer and burning of the coil.

• As the ammeter is always connected in series in the circuit, the resistance of an ideal ammeter should be zero. Hence, a low resistance is connected in parallel to the galvanometer, so that the resultant resistance becomes very low and almost all the currents pass through the galvanometer.

Features of an Ammeter

1. It is used to measure electrical current flowing in an electrical circuit.

2. It is always connected in series with an electrical circuit.

3. A low resistance is connected in parallel with its coil. An ideal ammeter has zero resistance.

OSCILLOSCOPES

Oscilloscopes (7 Marks)

The oscilloscope, or scope for short, is a device for drawing calibrated graphs of voltage *vs* time very quickly and conveniently. Such an instrument is obviously useful for the design and repair of circuits in which voltages and currents are changing with time (Fig. 6.37).

There are two types of oscilloscopes: *Analog* and *digital*.

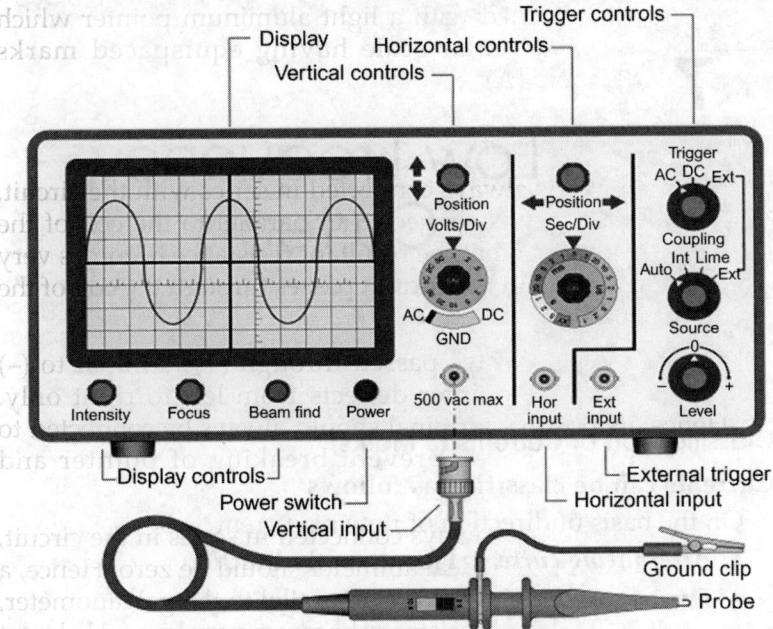

Fig. 6.37: Oscilloscope

Analog oscilloscopes use a cathode ray tube and display the signal much like a television set displays an image.

Digital oscilloscopes sample the signals digitally and are more flexible in how they display, manipulate, and store the signals.

The heart of the oscilloscope is a cathode ray tube or CRT. Electronic circuits in the scope apply voltages to one set of deflection plates to sweep the beam across the screen from left to right at a constant rate, thereby providing the time axis.

Other circuits amplify or attenuate the input signal as needed, and apply voltages to the other set of deflection plates to move the beam vertically, providing the voltage axis. Controls are provided to select the time and voltage scales needed for any given situation.

Low Frequency Currents

Classification of Currents (3 Marks)

Currents can be classified as follows

1. On the basis of direction of flow of current
   - *Alternating current*: Flow in both direction
   - *Direct current*: Flow in one direction
2. On the basis of frequency
   - *Low frequency currents*: Ranges from 01 to 1000 Hz, e.g. faradic, galvanic, sinusoidal, TENS
   - *Medium frequency currents*: Range of 1000 to 10,000 Hz, e.g. IFT, Russian currents
   - *High frequency currents*: Frequency more than 1 MHz, e.g. SWD, MWD, ultrasound therapy.
3. On the basis of voltage
   - *Low voltage currents*: Less than 100 volt
   - *High voltage currents*: Greater than 100 volt
4. On the basis of amperage
   - *Low amperage currents*: 1 to 30 mA, e.g. high TENS
   - *High amperage currents*: 500 to 2000 mA

Direct Current and Interrupted Direct Current (3 Marks)

Direct current: This is electric current whose direction of polarity is constant and passes continuously in one direction only (Fig. 7.1).

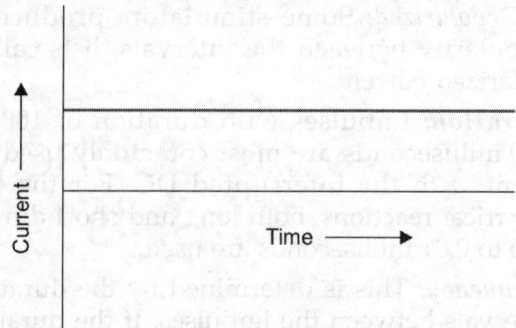

Fig. 7.1: Direct current

Interrupted direct current: Interruption is the most usual modification of the direct current. It makes the flow of current commence and cease at regular intervals (Fig. 7.2).

Various types of impulses are available with the interrupted DC, depending on the following factors:

I. *Waveform*

1. *Rectangular:* When there is sudden rise, short stay at peak and sudden fall in the impulse.
2. *Trapezoidal:* When there is gradual rise and fall of impulse with a short stay at peak.
3. *Triangular:* When there is sudden rise and fall of the impulse with no stay at the peak.
4. *Saw-tooth:* When there is very gradual rise but sudden fall of the impulse.

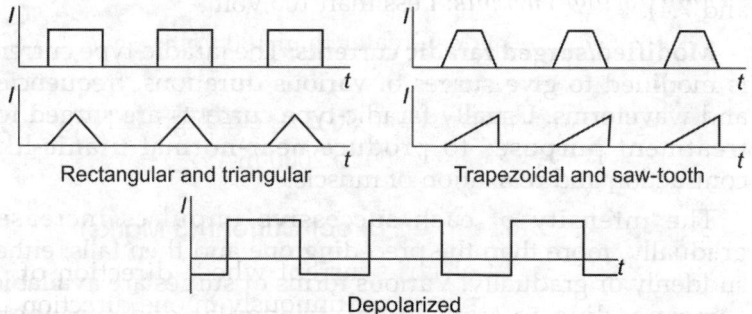

Rectangular and triangular   Trapezoidal and saw-tooth

Depolarized

Fig. 7.2: Interrupted direct current

5. *Depolarized:* Some stimulators produce reversal polarity between the intervals, it is called depolarized current.

II. **Duration:** Impulses with duration of 100, 300 and 600 milliseconds are most commonly used for treatment with the interrupted DC. For the testing of electrical reactions, both long and short durations, i.e. 100 to 0.01 milliseconds are used.

III. **Frequency:** This is determined by the duration of the intervals between the impulses. If the duration of the impulse is increased the frequency should be reduced. Usually 30 impulses per minute is suitable for interrupted DC treatment with duration of 100 milliseconds.

IV. **Depolarization:** A current of low intensity may flow in the reverse direction during the interval between the impulses. The chemical formation which accompanies the passage of a DC through an electrolyte is reduced by depolarized current.

Faradic-type Current and Surged Faradic Currents (3 Marks)

Faradic-type current: A faradic-type current is a short-duration interrupted direct current with pulse duration of 0.1–1 ms and frequency of 50–100 Hz.

The term 'Faradism' was originally used to the current as it is produced by faradic coil. The current provided by the first faradic coil was an unevenly alternating current but now the faradic coils are suppressed by electronic stimulators (Figs 7.3 and 7.4).

Modified/surged faradic currents: The faradic-type current is modified to give surges of various durations, frequencies and waveforms. Usually faradic-type currents are surged for treatment purposes to produce near-normal titanic-like contraction and relaxation of muscle.

The intensity of each successive impulses increases gradually, more than the preceding one and then falls, either suddenly or gradually. Various forms of surges are available, corresponding to trapezoidal, triangular and saw-tooth impulses (Fig. 7.5).

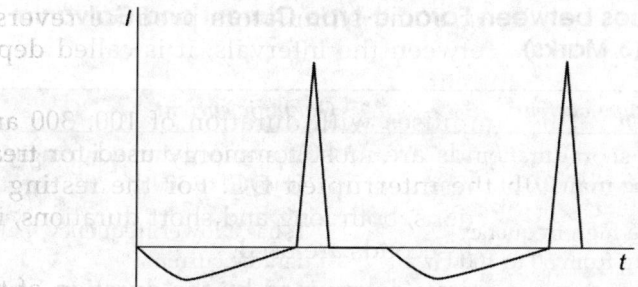

Fig. 7.3: Original faradic current

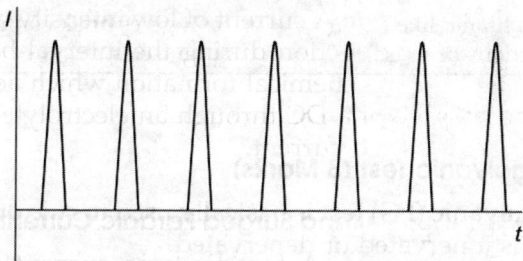

Fig. 7.4: Modern faradic current

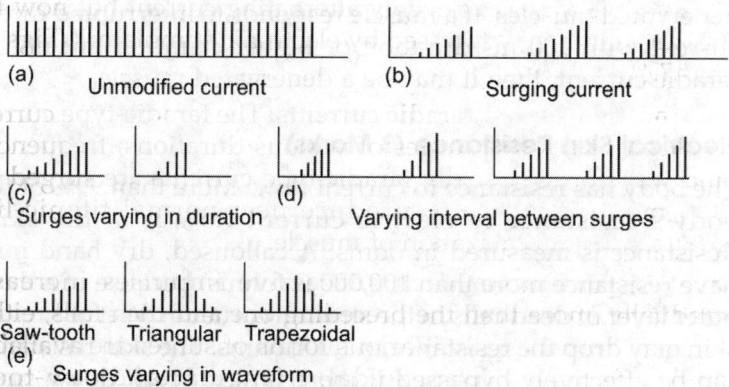

(a) Unmodified current

(b) Surging current

(c) Surges varying in duration

(d) Varying interval between surges

Saw-tooth   Triangular   Trapezoidal

(e) Surges varying in waveform

Fig. 7.5a to e: Modified/surged faradic currents

Differences between Faradic-type Current and Galvanic Current (3 Marks)

Faradic-type current	Galvanic current
1. It is of short duration ranging from 0.01 to 1 ms	1. It is of long duration ranging from 10 to 300 ms
2. It has a high frequency ranging from 50 to 100 Hz	2. It has a lower frequency than faradic current
3. It is used to stimulate innervated muscles	3. It is used to stimulate denervated muscles
4. It gives mild prickling type of sensation	4. It gives stabbing type of sensation
5. It gives titanic-like contractions of muscles	5. It gives brisk contraction of muscles

Faradic-galvanic Test (3 Marks)

Faradic-galvanic (FG) test is basically used to rule out whether a muscle is innervated or denervated.

Pertaining to characteristics of faradic current, i.e. pulse duration 0.01–1 ms and frequency 50–100 Hz, it will stimulate only innervated muscles and not denervated muscles. Whereas interrupted direct current with pulse duration such as 100 ms or 300 ms will stimulate both innervated and denervated muscles. If a muscle responds to interrupted direct current with 100 ms duration or higher duration but not to faradic current, then it may be a denervated muscle.

Electrical Skin Resistance (3 Marks)

The body has resistance to current flow. More than 99% of the body's resistance to electric current flow is at the skin. Resistance is measured in ohms. A calloused, dry hand may have resistance more than 100,000 Ω (ohms) because of a thick outer layer of dead cells in the stratum corneum. Wet or broken skin may drop the resistance to 1,000 ohms. The skin resistance can be effectively bypassed if there is skin break down from high voltage, a cut, a deep abrasion, or immersion in water.

Skin resistance can be greatly reduced by the following ways

1. Moisten electrodes with water or gel
2. Remove dirt, oil, or flaky skin by washing area
3. Warm area with moist heat pack
4. Remove excessive hair
5. Saturate sponge with saline solution instead of water
6. Immersion in water (water bath method)

Types of Electrodes (7 Marks)

There are number of different electrodes that is used in the clinical setting. Each type has certain advantages and disadvantages.

A variety of electrodes that is commonly used:

Carbon-rubber electrodes: These are probably the most commonly used electrodes in clinical setting. They comes in a variety of sizes and usually black and red (Fig. 7.6). These electrodes are either used with moistened sponge or electrolytic gel placed between them and the patient's skin.

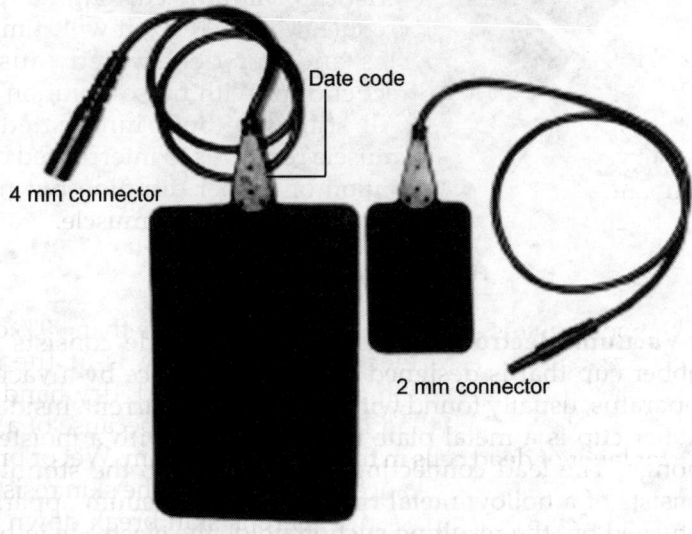

Fig. 7.6: Carbon-rubber electrodes

The rubber electrodes must be held in firm contact with the skin, this is usually accomplished by the use of elastic straps.

The advantages of this type of electrode include ease of use, pliability, and availability. Disadvantages include that they tend to get dirty and become less pliable with age, when sponges are used with these electrodes, they should be disinfected between each patient application.

Metal plate electrodes: These types of electrodes are less frequently used nowadays. They come in a variety of shapes and sizes. These electrodes are used with moistened lint pad placed between them and the patient's skin. The lint pad should be of eight folds. As with rubber electrodes, metal electrodes must be held in place with some type of strap (Fig. 7.7).

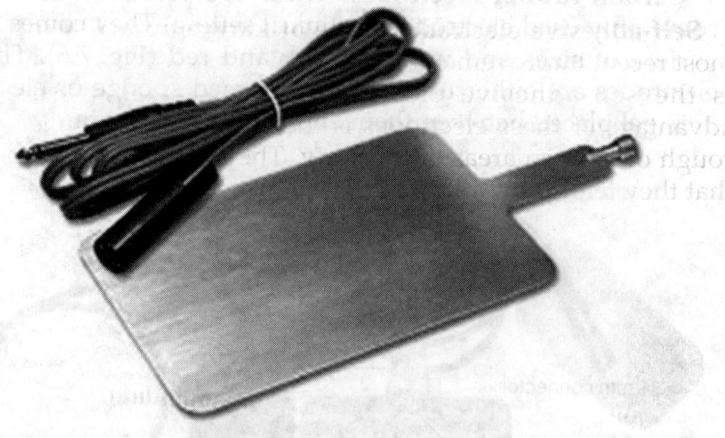

Fig. 7.7: Metal plate electrode

Vacuum electrodes: This type of electrode consists of a rubber cup that is designed to be held in place by a vacuum apparatus, usually found with interferential current. Inside the rubber cup is a metal plate that is covered with a moistened sponge. The lead connecting the electrode to the stimulator consists of a hollow metal ring. When the vacuum apparatus is turned on, the resulting suction holds the electrode in place (Fig. 7.8).

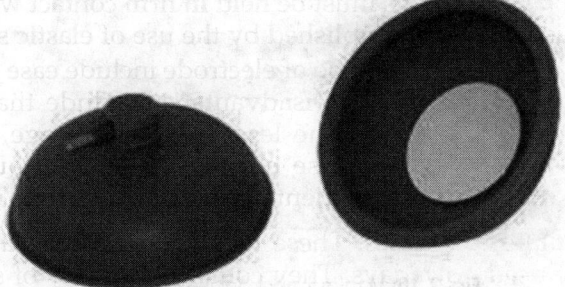

Fig. 7.8: Vacuum electrodes

The primary advantage of these electrodes is the ability to apply them in rough or uneven areas of the body. Disadvantages include the creation of a welt under the electrode and the added expense of the vacuum apparatus.

Self-adhesive electrodes made of karaya gum: One of the most recent improvements in the field of electrical stimulation is the self-adhesive electrodes (Fig. 7.9). The primary advantage of these electrodes is the ability to apply them in rough or uneven areas of the body. The only disadvantage is that they tend to wear out after repeated use.

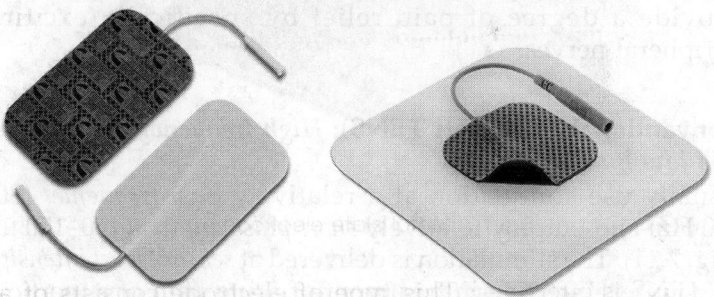

Fig. 7.9: Self-adhesive electrodes

Intra-vaginal or intra-anal electrodes: *Electrical stimulation can be used* to treat *urinary incontinence*. The device consists of a plastic probe with two embedded ring electrodes. The small *electrical* impulses are delivered to the *pelvic* structures through an internal *vaginal* or *anal electrode* (Fig. 7.10).

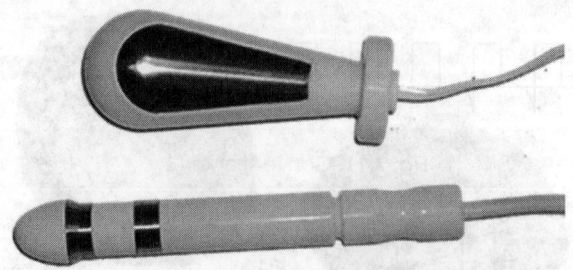

Fig. 7.10: Vaginal and anal electrodes

Transvaginal electrical stimulation (TVES) is the non-painful application of electrical current using a sensor with electrodes placed in the vagina to directly stimulate the pelvic floor muscles to contract and relax. Male patients suffering from incontinence following prostatectomy may be treated by using a rectal electrode.

Types of TENS (7 Marks)

Transcutaneous electrical nerve stimulation (TENS): It is a non-invasive method of electrical stimulation via surface electrodes on the patient's intact skin and primarily aims to provide a degree of pain relief by specifically exciting peripheral nerves.

Conventional TENS (Hi TENS): *High frequency, short pulse and low intensity*
Usually use stimulation at a relatively *high frequency* (80–150 Hz) and employ relatively *short pulse duration* (50–150 µs) (Fig. 7.11). The stimulation is delivered at *sensory level intensity*. Hi TENS is effective in treatment of acute pain of superficial nature.

Acupuncture (low) TENS: *Low frequency, relatively long pulse and high intensity*
Use stimulation at low frequency (2–5 Hz) with long pulse duration (150–250 µs). The stimulation is delivered at motor level intensity (Fig. 7.12). As it provokes visible muscle

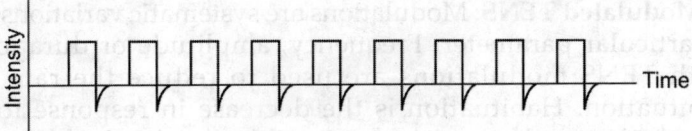

Fig. 7.11: Conventional TENS

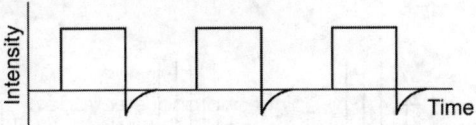

Fig. 7.12: Acupuncture TENS

contraction. Low TENS is effective in treatment of chronic pain of damaged deep tissues.

Burst TENS: *High frequency, short pulse and high intensity in 'trains'*

It is conventional TENS (Fig. 7.13), but delivered in the burst mode therefore interrupting the stimulation outflow at the rate of 2–7 bursts/sec. Each burst consists of a number of individual pulses at high frequency and short pulse duration as conventional TENS but with high stimulation intensity and burst duration is 300–1000 μs. For some patients this is by far the most effective approach to pain relief.

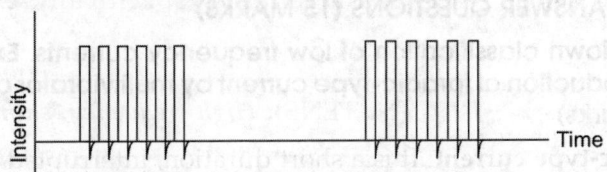

Fig. 7.13: Burst TENS

Brief intense TENS: This is a TENS mode that can be employed to achieve a rapid pain relief, but some patients may find the strength of the stimulation too intense. The pulse frequency applied is high (120–250 Hz band) and the pulse width is also high (200–250 μs plus).

The current is delivered at, or close to the tolerance level for the patient, such that they would not want the machine turned up any higher.

Modulated TENS: Modulations are systematic variations in a particular parameter: Frequency, amplitude or duration. With TENS modulations are used to reduce the rate of habituation. Habituation is the decrease in response to a repeated stimulus and is responsible for the decrease in perception of a sensory stimulus (Fig. 7.14).

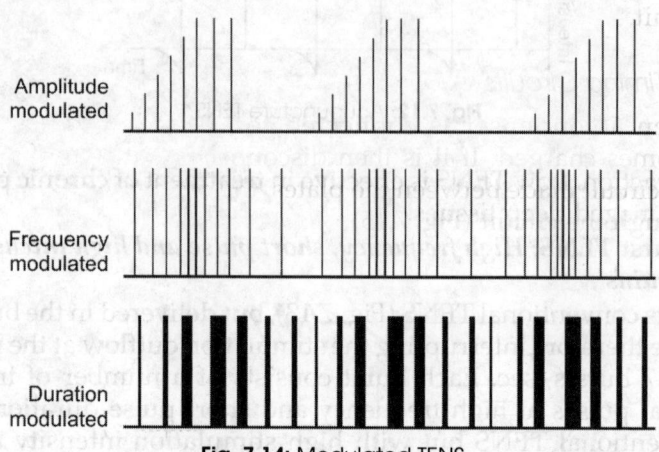

Fig. 7.14: Modulated TENS

LONG ANSWER QUESTIONS (15 MARKS)

Write down classification of low frequency currents. Explain the production of faradic-type current by multivibrator circuit. (15 Marks)

Faradic-type current: It is a short duration, interrupted direct current, with pulse duration of 0.1 to 1 ms and a frequency of 50 to 100 Hz.

Production of faradic-type currents: The faradic type current is produced by the modern electronic stimulators containing a circuit called the multivibrator circuit.

The principles underlying working of the circuit are
- The switching action of the triode valves
- The working of the CR timing circuit
- Wiring of resistances in series

Switching Action of the Triode Valve

When a triode valve is connected into a circuit, the filament is heated and current passes across the valve. The grid lies between the filament and the anode. If a sufficiently strong negative charge is applied to the grid the current across the valve ceases, while if the grid loses this negative charge the current flows again, thus the valve can act as a switch in the circuit.

CR Timing Circuits

When a condenser is connected to a source of supply it becomes charged. If it is then disconnected from the supply and circuit made between the plates, the condenser discharges through the circuit (Fig. 7.15).

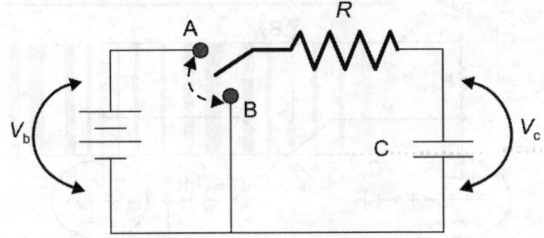

Fig. 7.15: CR timing circuit

When the switch is in position A the condenser is charged from the cell. When the switch is moved to position B the condenser discharges through the resistance. The time taken for the condenser to discharge depends on the capacity of the condenser and the resistance of the circuit.

The duration of the condenser discharge varies with $C \times R$

Where C = Capacity of the condenser (farad)

R = Resistance of the circuit (ohms)

Resistances in Series

When resistances are wired in series with each other the potential drop across each is directly proportional to its resistance.

If two equal resistances (R_1 and R_2) are wired in series with each other and PD of 100 volts is applied to the circuit, there is PD of 50 volts across each resistance as each is half the total resistance of the circuit.

Wiring of multivibrator circuit

- The circuit consists of two triode valves (V_1, V_2) are wired in parallel to each other between the supply lines.
- A resistance is placed between each anode and the positive supply line (Ra_1, Ra_2) which are wired in series with valves V_1 and V_2.
- In parallel with each valve is a condenser and a resistance, in series with each other (C_1R_1, C_2R_2).
- One plate of each condenser is connected to the anode of one valve (A_1, A_2) and other to the grid of the other valves (G_2, G_1) and resistances (R_1, R_2) (Fig. 7.16).

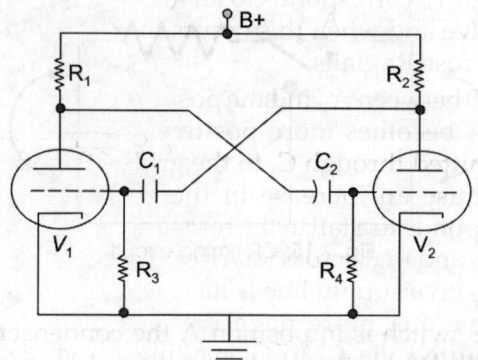

Fig. 7.16a: Schematic view

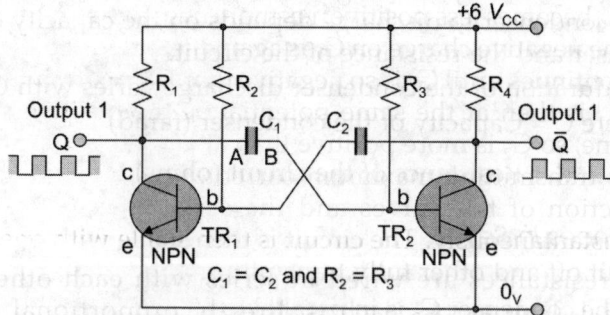

Fig. 7.16b: Wiring of multivibrator circuit

Note: Transistors are used in preference to the valves, in most modern electrical stimulators, as they are durable, have a long life, consume less power and need no heating device.

Working of multivibrator circuit: When the current is first switched on it passes equally across both valves but a circuit of this type is very sensitive to interference from outside sources. Rise or fall in the intensity of the current flowing through either valve because of interference initiates the action of the circuit.

If the change is a decrease in the intensity of current across V_1 the following sequence of events takes place:

- In accordance with the principles of resistances in series, the potential drop between the supply lines is divided between V_1 and Ra_1 in direct proportion to their resistance. A decrease in the intensity of the current passing through V_1 corresponds to an increase in the resistance of the valve and when this occurs the PD across it rises and that across Ra_1 falls.

- The PD between A_1 and the positive supply line is reduced and A_1 becomes more positive. The positive charge is transmitted through C_1 to the grid of the other valve (G_2) and cause an increase in the current across V_2. This corresponds to a fall in the resistance of V_2 so the PD across V_2 falls and that across Ra_2 rises. Thus, PD between A_2 and the positive supply line is increased and A_2 becomes less positive, i.e. more negative. The negative charge is transmitted via C_2 to G_1 making it more negative and further reducing the intensity of the current across V_1.

- A_2 becomes less positive, i.e. more negative and therefore, the negative charge on G_1 is again increased. This process continues until G_1 is so negative that V_1 ceases to conduct. A_1 is then at the same potential as the positive supply line, so G_2 is more positive than at any other time and V_2 is transmitting maximum current. This is the switching action of the valves and the series of events occurs instantaneously. The circuit is then stable with one valve cut off and other fully transmitting.

- The condenser C_2 is in parallel to V_2 and so the PD across it is the same as that across the valve. C_2 is charged at the beginning, the left hand plate being negative and the right hand plate positive. During the above sequence PD across V_2 falls and so that across C_2 also falls. C_2 therefore begins to discharge through R_2 and V_2 and its left hand plate gradually loses its negative charge.

- The grid of V_1 is connected to this plate, therefore as the condenser discharges G_1 also loses its negative charge. When the charge falls to a certain level V_1 again begins to transmit current. The time that elapses before this occurs depends on the duration of the condenser discharge which is determined by the product of the capacity of C_2 and the ohmic resistance of R_2, i.e. $(C_2 \times R_2)$.

- When V_1 begins to transmit current the switching action is again brought into play but acting in the reverse direction to the previous one. Consequently V_2 is cut off and V_1 transmits maximum current. This state lasts until the discharge of C_1 through R_1. Thus, the current passes first through one valve then through the other. The duration of flow through V_2 during which V_1 is cut off depends on C_2R_2, whereas the duration of flow through V_1 during which V_2 is cut off depends on C_1R_1.

Current supplied to the patient

- The patient circuit is wired in parallel to Ra_2 and the interrupted current which flows through this resistance is also supplied to the patient. The periods of current flow occur when V_2 is transmitting and their duration is determined by C_2R_2. The interval occurs when V_2 is cut off and their duration is determined by C_1R_1.

- By using variable resistances for R_2 and R_1 the duration and frequency of the impulses can be adjusted. Increase in the resistance of R_2 increases the duration of the stimuli, while increase in the resistance of R1 increases the intervals between them and so reduces their frequency.

- The resistances may be varied either by using a series rheostat or by moving a switch so that a different resistance coil is included. Either method can be used for each resistance or may be observed in different apparatus.

Medium Frequency Currents

SHORT ANSWER QUESTIONS

Beat Frequency (3 Marks)

* Interferential therapy utilizes two medium frequency currents which pass through the tissues simultaneously. They are set up so that their paths cross; and in simple terms they interfere with each other. This interference gives rise to *interference current or beat frequency* (Fig. 8.1), which has the characteristics of low-frequency stimulation.

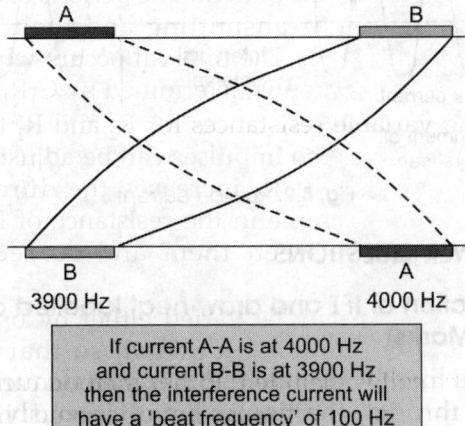

A   B

B   A
3900 Hz   4000 Hz

If current A-A is at 4000 Hz
and current B-B is at 3900 Hz
then the interference current will
have a 'beat frequency' of 100 Hz

Fig. 8.1: Beat frequency

93

- The exact frequency of the resultant beat frequency can be controlled by the input frequencies. For example, if one current was at 4000 Hz and the other current at 3900 Hz, the resultant beat frequency would be at 100 Hz.

Russian Current (3 Marks)

- Russian current is 2.5 kHz alternating current delivered in sinusoidal or rectangular bursts with a burst frequency of 50 Hz and pulse varies from 50 to 250 μs; the phase duration is half of the pulse duration or 25–125 μs, i.e. 50% duty cycle (Fig. 8.2).
- Russian current is applied in trains of bursts with a '10/50/ 10' treatment application. The bursts of current are applied for 10 sec followed by a 50 sec rest period and the stimulation is repeated for 10 minutes of treatment.
- To make intensity of current tolerable it is generated in 50-burst per second envelopes with an interburst interval of 10 ms.
- The main clinical uses of Russian current are for obtaining a motor response, specifically for muscle contraction and strengthening.

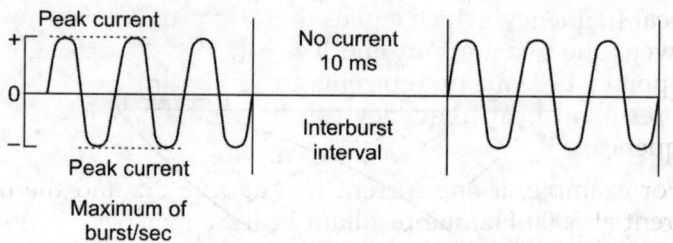

Fig. 8.2: Russian current

LONG ANSWER QUESTIONS

Write production of IFT and draw neat labelled diagram of IFT unit (15 Marks)

Interferential therapy utilizes two medium frequency currents which pass through the tissues simultaneously to interfere with each other. This interference gives rise to *beat frequency*, which has characteristics of low-frequency stimulation.

PRINCIPLE OF PRODUCTION OF IFT

Continuous interference: When two waves slightly out of phase collide and form a single wave with progressively increasing and decreasing amplitude (Fig. 8.3).

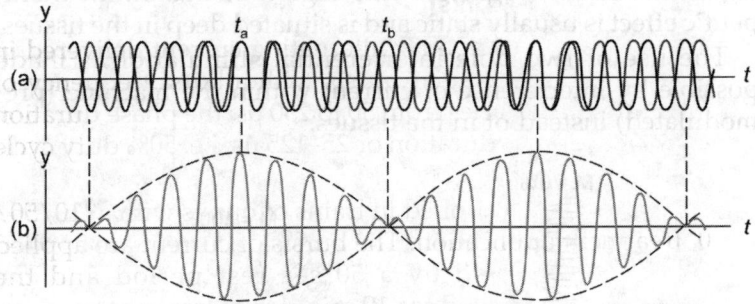

Fig. 8.3: Continuous interference

Production of Interferential Current (IFC)

One of the median frequency currents is kept at a constant frequency of 4000 Hz and the other can be varied between 3900 to 4000 Hz. An interference of these two frequencies results in a 'beat frequency' which equals to the difference in frequency between the two currents and it is produced in the tissues at the point where the two currents cross. The exact frequency of the resultant beat frequency can be controlled by the input frequencies.

For example, if one current was at 4000 Hz and the other current at 3900 Hz, the resultant beat frequency would be at 100 Hz (*refer* to Fig. 8.1).

Four electrodes are used in two pairs, each pair being indicated by the coloring of the wire from the machine. The electrodes of each pair are placed diagonally opposite one another in such a way that the interference effect or beat frequency is produced in the tissues where it is required. Variations in the interference frequencies can be pre-selected on the machine and may be constant and rhythmic. A 'rhythmic mode' indicates that the frequency is swinging continuously from the lower to the higher value and back.

The beat frequency current flows maximally in the region of maximum interference that develops along diagonals extending at 45° to the direct path between the two sets of electrodes. A clover leaf pattern of field is created, because one current flows laterally from its direct path to interact with the adjacent current (Fig. 8.4). This region of maximum therapeutic effect is usually static and is situated deep in the tissues.

The use of two pole interferential stimulation is made possible by interference of current within the machine (premodulated) instead of in the tissues.

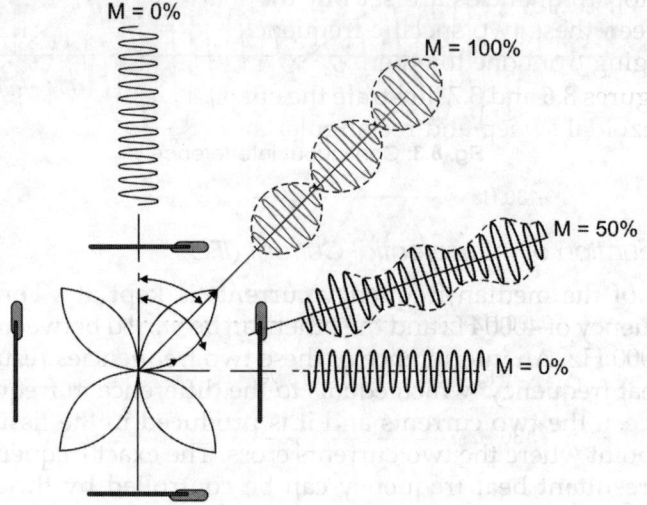

Fig. 8.4: Clover leaf pattern

Frequency Sweep

Nerves will accommodate to a constant signal and a sweep (gradually changing frequency) is often used to overcome this problem. The principle of using the sweep is that the machine is set to automatically vary the effective stimulation frequency using either pre-set or user set sweep ranges. The pattern of the sweep makes a significant difference to the stimulation received by the patient (Fig. 8.5). In the classic 'triangular' sweep pattern, the machine gradually changes from the base to the top frequency, usually over a time period of 6 seconds.

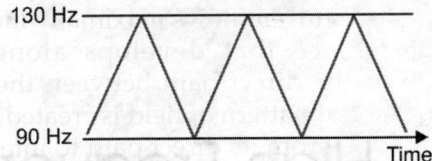

Fig. 8.5: Triangular sweep pattern

Other patterns of sweep can be produced on many machines, e.g. a 'rectangular' sweep and the 'trapezoidal' sweep pattern produces a very different stimulation pattern in that the base and top frequencies are set but the machine then 'switches' between these two specific frequencies rather than gradually changing from one to other.

Figures 8.6 and 8.7 illustrate the effect of setting a 90–130 Hz trapezoidal sweep and rectangular sweep.

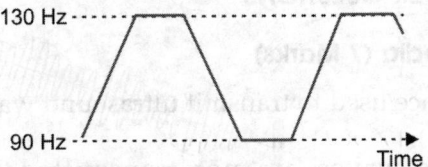

Fig. 8.6: Trapezoidal sweep pattern

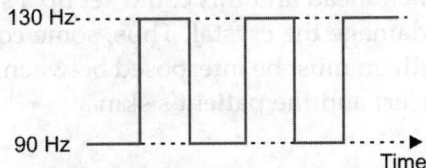

Fig. 8.7: Rectangular sweep pattern

High Frequency Currents

SHORT ANSWER QUESTIONS

Coupling Media (7 Marks)

It is a substance used to transmit ultrasound waves to tissues.

Ultrasonic waves are not transmitted by air (zero transmission). Air will in fact reflect the ultrasonic beam back into the treatment head and this could set up a standing wave which might damage the crystal. Thus, some couplant which does transmit them must be interposed between the treatment head (transducer) and the patient's skin.

Properties of coupling media are as follows

- It must be viscous enough to fill cavities between transducer and skin.

- Air interface must be minimized

- It must not be readily absorbed by the skin

- It must have acoustic impedance similar to human tissue

- It should necessarily prevent undue reflection and absorption.

Efficiency of transmission of ultrasound by various coupling media

Couplant	% Transmission
Aquasonic gel	72.6
Glycerol	67
Distilled water	59
Liquid paraffin	19
Petroleum jelly	0
Air	0

LONG ANSWER QUESTIONS (15 MARKS)

1. Describe the production of ultrasound. Draw a panel diagram of ultrasound. (15 Marks) (Summer 2017)
2. Write in detail production of ultrasound and methods of testing the apparatus.

Ultrasound: Ultrasound refers to mechanical vibrations, which are essentially the same as sound waves but has a frequency higher than audible frequency limit of human hearing (i.e. >20,000 Hz). Therapeutic frequencies are being in the region of 1 MHz or 3 MHz.

PRINCIPLE OF PRODUCTION

Direct piezoelectric effect: Generation of electrical impulse when piezoelectric crystal is compressed is known as direct piezoelectric effect (Fig. 9.1).

Expanded voltage of opposite polarity is generated, which converts ultrasound beam to electrical energy that replicate sound pattern.

Reverse piezoelectric effect: Contraction and expansion of piezoelectric crystal in response to voltage across it is known as reverse piezoelectric effect (Fig. 9.2).

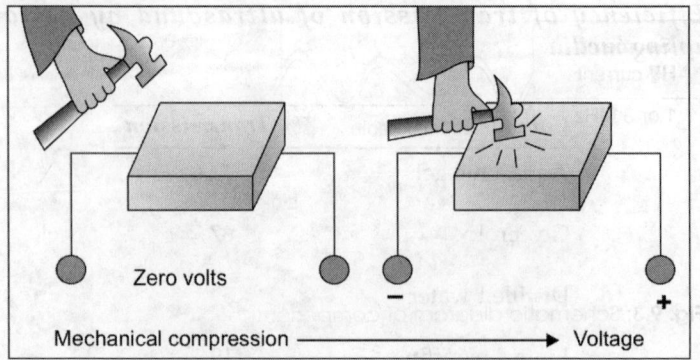

Fig. 9.1: Direct piezoelectric effect

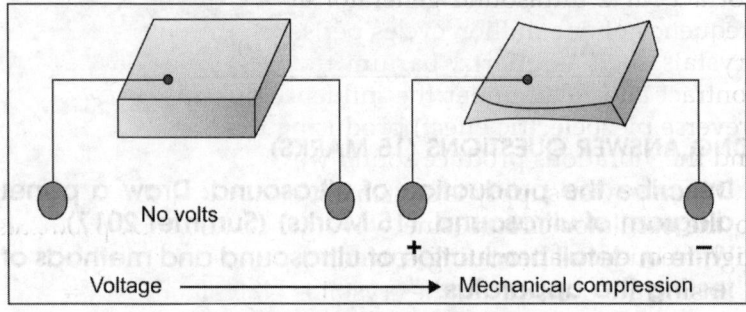

Fig. 9.2: Reverse piezoelectric effect

The crystal vibrates at frequency of electrical signal.

All therapeutic ultrasound generators are constructed on the reverse piezoelectric principle.

Components of Ultrasonic Apparatus

Source of supply: A source of high-frequency current is conveyed by a coaxial cable to a transducer circuit or treatment head.

Transducer circuit: The high-frequency current is applied to the crystal via a linking electrode. The crystal is fused to the metal front plate of the treatment head and the linking electrode.

Figure 9.3 shows the schematic diagram of components of ultrasound apparatus.

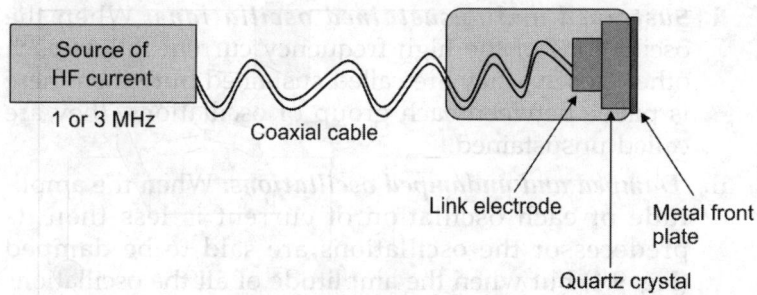

Fig. 9.3: Schematic diagram of components of ultrasound apparatus

PRODUCTION OF ULTRASOUND

For a 1 MHz ultrasound generator a vibrating source with a frequency of one million cycles per second is needed. Certain crystals such as quartz, barium titanate, zinc titanate, etc. contract and relax under the influence of an electric current (reverse piezoelectric effect) producing mechanical vibrations and the vibrations produce sound waves.

When power supply is switch on, electrical energy is given to the oscillator circuit (sine wave generator), that produces high-frequency alternating current.

Inside the transducer, the crystal is embedded between the link electrode and the metal front plate. The crystal being fused to the link electrode, responds to high-frequency current that is fed through the coaxial cable. The crystal contracts and expands at the same frequency at which the current changes polarity.

Any change in the shape of the crystal causes a movement of the metal front plate which in turn produces an ultrasonic wave. The current applied to the oscillator circuit can be automatically made on and off to give pulse output.

SHORT WAVE DIATHERMY

SHORT ANSWER QUESTIONS

1. Properties of High Frequency Currents (3 Marks)

A high frequency current has a frequency of more than 10,000 Hz. It exhibits certain properties which are as follows:

i. *Sustained and unsustained oscillations:* When the oscillations of the high frequency current follow each other closely, they are called sustained but when there is pause between each group of oscillations, they are called unsustained.

ii. *Damped and undamped oscillations:* When the amplitude of each oscillation of current is less than its predecessor the oscillations are said to be damped (Fig. 9.4) but when the amplitude of all the oscillations is same they are called undamped (Fig. 9.5).

iii. *Heat production:* High frequency currents produce heat, like other currents in accordance with Joule's law.

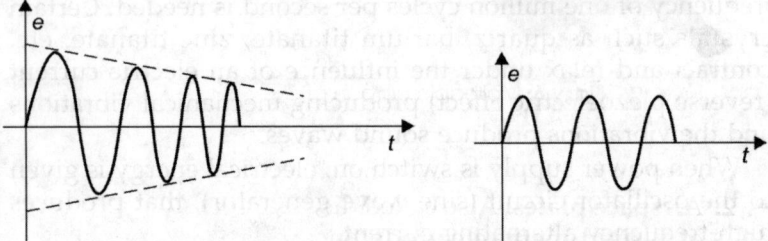

Fig. 9.4: Damped oscillations   **Fig. 9.5:** Undamped and sustained oscillations

2. Indicators of Tuning of SWD Machine (3 Marks)

i. An ammeter/galvanometer wired in the circuit shows maximum reading that diminishes by turning the knob.

ii. A neon lamp attached with the machine glows maximally when the tuning knob is moved.

iii. A tube containing a small amount of neon gas placed within the electric field between the electrodes will glow at maximum intensity when the circuits are in resonance.

3. Types of Electrodes (7 Marks)

There are various types of capacitor electrodes, but each consists of a metal plate surrounded by some form of insulating material.

1. **Malleable/flexible pad:** It consists of a malleable metal plate encased in rubber and produces an electrostatic field. This can be moulded to the body part, but should not be bent sharply or the metal plate may crack (Fig. 9.6).

   Electrodes of this type are separated from the skin by perforated felt, which is the most satisfactory spacing material.

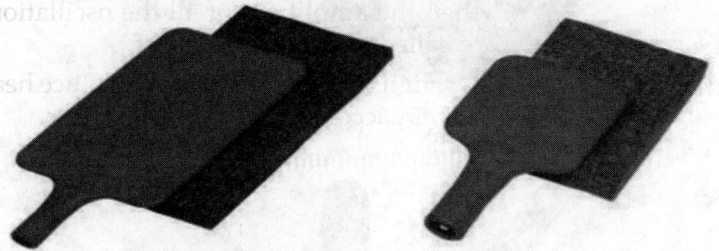

Fig. 9.6: Malleable carbon pad electrodes

2. **Airspace plates:** Also called disc electrodes. These consist of a rigid metal electrode encased in a Perspex cover within which the position of the metal plate can be adjusted. These electrodes are commonly circular (Fig. 9.7).

   Electrodes of this type are arranged in position on supporting arms and it is advisable to leave a small gap between the cover and the skin to allow for the circulation of air.

3. **The monode:** Also called drum electrode. This is a flat, rigid coil encased in plastic cover and produces an electromagnetic field (Fig. 9.8). These electrodes are arranged in position on supporting arms and are separated from the skin by an air gap.

4. **The diplode:** It consists of a flat coil electrode encased in a Perspex cover with two wings (Fig. 9.9). These electrodes are arranged in position on supporting arms and are separated from the skin by an air gap.

5. **Coil or cable electrodes:** The cable electrode consists of a thick wire covered with rubber and plugs at either end

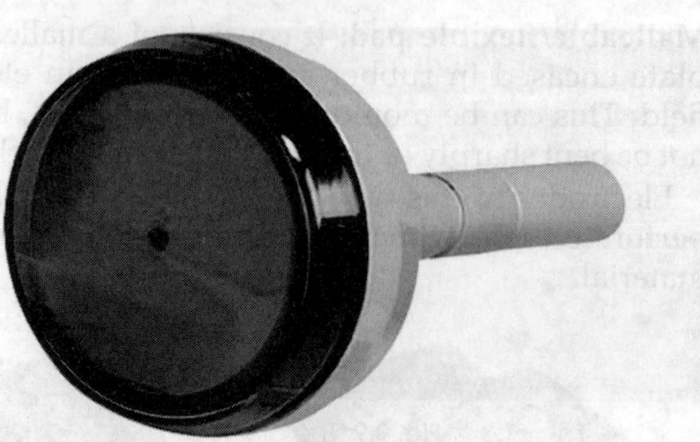

1. Method: A movable pad is supported by a metal plate around 3 in rubber with the two electrode and hold. The capacity plate itself but should not packed shut, but it is for discharge of the most common but this also by particular distance which is within material.

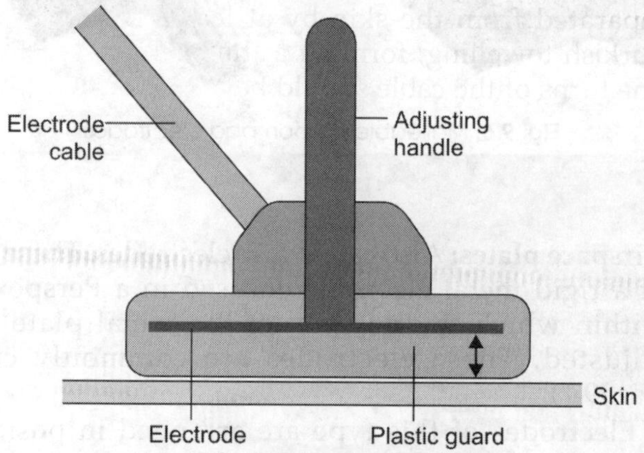

the electrode plate as plate above sheath with separated through.

2. Airspace plates:
were width within a satisfied.

3. Electrode plates: type are small. In this air on appropriate, and it is advisable to leave a small gap between probe and the skin. The skin itself or the air between the probe and skin offers the capacitation the motode. Also called drum electrode. This is then

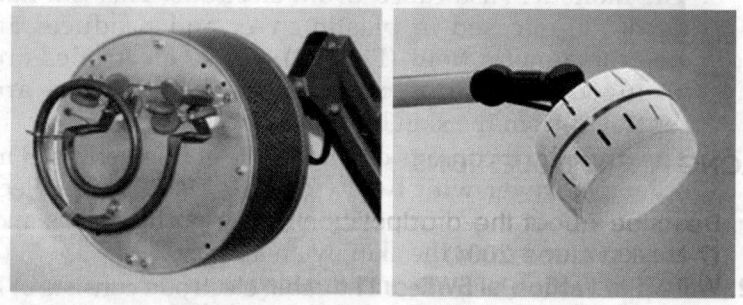

Fig. 9.7a and b: Airspace plates (disc electrode)

Fig. 9.8: The monode (drum electrode)

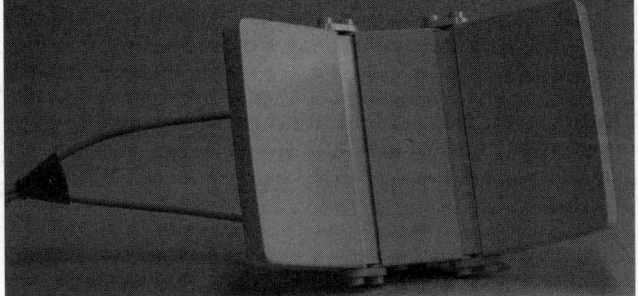

Fig. 9.9: The diplode

(Fig. 9.10). It produces electromagnetic field. It is separated from the skin by at least four layers of dry Turkish towelling, forming a thickness of at least 1 cm. The turns of the cable should be at least 2.5 cm apart.

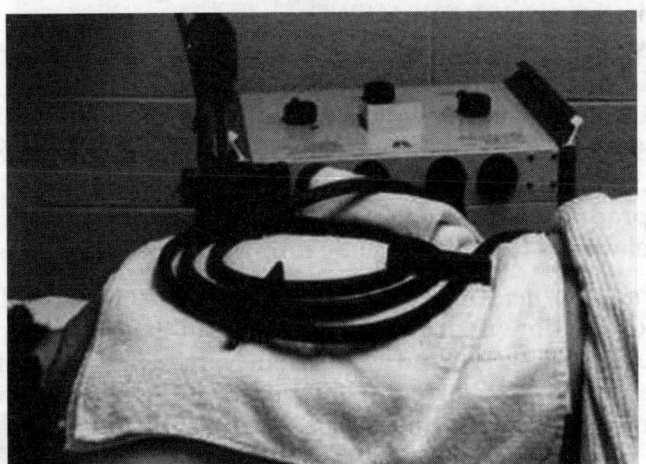

Fig. 9.10: Cable electrode

LONG ANSWER QUESTIONS

1. Describe about the production of short wave diathermy. (7 Marks) (June 2004)
2. Write production of SWD and draw neat labelled diagram of SWD unit. (15 Marks)

Components of SWD Machine

There are two circuits in SWD machine: Oscillator circuit and resonator circuit.

Oscillator circuit: It is also called machine circuit. The high frequency current is generated by this circuit at a precise frequency of 27.12 MHz and the wavelength of 11 meters. It consists of:

   i. Mains supply
  ii. Transformers (step-up and step-down)
 iii. Triode valve
 iv. Grid leak resistance
  v. Oscillator coil

Mains supply: It is connected with AC mains that give 240 volts and frequency of 50 cycles/sec.

Transformers: There are two types of transformer which are used in the construction of SWD.

a. *Step-up transformer:* The secondary coil of this transformer is connected with the oscillator circuit, which in turn is connected with the triode valve.

b. *Step-down transformer:* The secondary coil of which is connected with the filament of the triode valve and produces a potential of 20 volts, which cause emission of electrons from the cathode through thermionic emission.

Triode valve: This is a thermionic valve, which allows electrons to flow in one direction, i.e. from the cathode to the anode (Fig. 9.11). The grid of the triode valve acts as a regulator to the flow of the current, i.e. when positive allows flow of current and when negative stops the current flow.

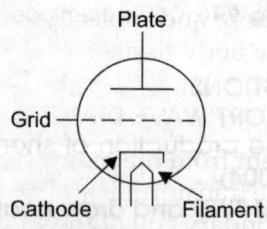

Fig. 9.11: Triode valve

Grid leak resistance: It consists of a resistance coil connected to the grid of the triode valve at one end and the filament of the cathode at the other.

Oscillator coil: It consists of a stable condenser and an oscillator coil, which gives high magnitude, high frequency oscillating currents to the resonator circuit.

Resonator circuit: It is also called patient's circuit, which lies parallel to the oscillator circuit. It consists of:

   i. Resonator coil
   ii. Variable condenser
   iii. Electrodes
   iv. Ammeter
   v. Tissue

Resonator coil: The high frequency and high magnitude current from the oscillator, flows in the resonator coil by electromagnetic induction.

Variable condenser: It is used for tuning the oscillator and the resonator circuit for having maximum transfer of energy to the patient through resonance.

Electrodes: The output of the SWD machine is connected to the electrodes which are positioned on the body tissue to be treated. Different types of electrodes are: Pad electrodes, disc electrodes, cable electrodes.

Ammeter: This shows maximum reading when the machine circuit and the patient's circuit resonate.

Tissue: This part of the body between the two electrodes form the dielectric of a condenser, where charges concentrate due to electrostatic field, to effect the tissues by causing dipole rotation, ionic vibration, and molecular distortion and hence producing heat in the body tissue.

PRODUCTION OF SHORT WAVE DIATHERMY

The alternating current from the mains supply passes through the primary coil of the transformer and an EMF of 20 to 25 volts is induced in the secondary coil of the step-down transformer, which is connected to the filament circuit of the triode valve. The filament is heated and thermionic emission takes place at the cathode. Similarly, an EMF of 4000 volts is induced in the secondary coil of the step-up transformer, which is connected to the anode circuit of the triode valve.

The anode of the valve is positive relative to the filament, thus current from the cathode flows towards the anode and in turn flows through the oscillator circuit in the direction C to D and back to the transformer. As the current in the oscillator coil (CD) rises in intensity, an EMF is induced in the coil AB, electrons moving in the direction B to A (Lenz's law). These electrons move on the grid of the valve, producing negative charge on it, which stops the flow of current through triode valve. As the current flow stops in the triode valve, the intensity of current in CD falls resulting in production of self-induced EMF, which prolongs the current flow and charges the condenser XY with 'Y' plate negative and 'X' plate positive.

When the self-induced EMF dies away, the condenser discharges through the oscillator coil and the current flows from D to C. As CD is an inductance, this is the first wave of an oscillating discharge and self-induced EMF recharges the condenser with 'X' negative and 'Y' positive. The flow of

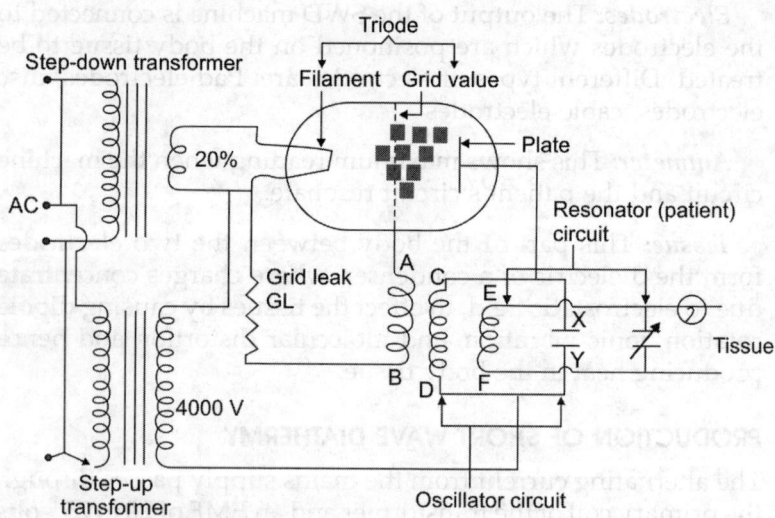

Fig. 9.12: Construction of short wave diathermy

current from D to C induces an EMF in AB, so that electrons start moving from A to B, causing the grid to lose its negative charge and restoring the flow of current in anode circuit. This cycle is repeated again and again, and in this way the oscillating current is produced in the oscillator circuit.

The resonator circuit is coupled with the oscillator circuit by inductors and a high frequency current is produced in it by electromagnetic induction. Maximum current flows in the patient (resonator) circuit when the oscillator circuit and the resonator circuit are in resonance (Fig. 9.12).

Actinotherapy

ELECTROMAGNETIC SPECTRUM AND LAWS GOVERNING RADIATION

1. Describe electromagnetic spectrum. Write laws governing radiation. (Nov-Dec 2009)
2. Explain with neat diagram various interactions of electromagnetic radiation with matter.
3. How the laws governing radiation are applicable for different modalities in physiotherapy?

Electromagnetic Spectrum

It is the distribution of electromagnetic radiation according to the energy or according to wavelength and frequency (Fig. 10.1).

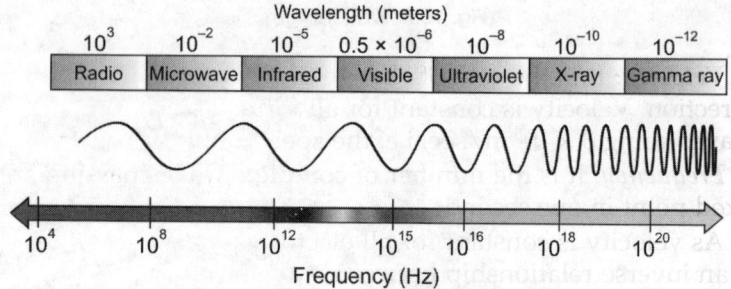

Fig. 10.1: Electromagnetic spectrum

Radio wave: 0.1 mm–100 km
Infrared: 750 nm–0.4 mm
Visible light: 400–750 nm

Ultraviolet: 10–400 nm
X-ray: 0.01 pm–100 nm
Gamma rays: 0.01–100 nm

Regions of Electromagnetic Spectrum

Ionizing range: Electromagnetic radiation such as X-ray and gamma rays is ionized radiation.

Non-ionizing range: Low frequency electromagnetic radiation is non-ionizing and cannot break molecular bonds or produce ions and so can be used for therapeutic medical applications. It includes visible light, ultraviolet rays, infrared rays, short wave and microwave.

The electromagnetic field is propagated by the interaction of alternating magnetic and electric field at right angle to one another.

Wavelength: Wavelength is the distance between a point on one electromagnetic wave and exactly the same point on the next wave (Fig. 10.2).

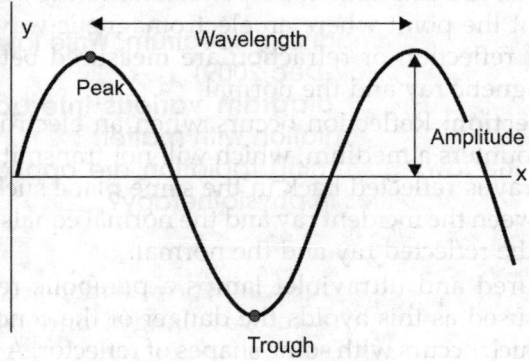

Fig. 10.2: Wavelength

Velocity: It is the rate of change of distance in a particular direction. Velocity is constant for all forms of electromagnetic waves being 3×10^8 m/sec, i.e. the speed of light.

Frequency: It is the number of complete waves passing any fixed point in one second.

As velocity is constant for all electromagnetic waves, there is an inverse relationship between wavelength and frequency for electromagnetic waves (Fig. 10.3).

Infrared, visible and ultraviolet waves travel in straight lines until they encounter a different medium when they may be transmitted, reflected or absorbed.

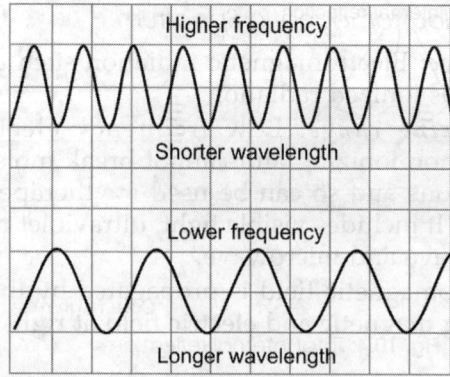

Fig. 10.3: Inverse relationship between wavelength and frequency

A normal is a line drawn perpendicular to the surface of a medium at the point where an electromagnetic wave strikes. Angles of reflection or refraction are measured between the electromagnetic ray and the normal.

1. Reflection: Reflection occurs when an electromagnetic wave encounters a medium, which will not transmit it. In this case, the ray is reflected back in the same plane such that the angle between the incident ray and the normal equals the angle between the reflected ray and the normal.

In infrared and ultraviolet lamps a parabolic reflector is normally used as this avoids the danger of the concentration of rays which occurs with some shapes of reflector. A parabolic reflector collects all the rays travelling in an inappropriate direction and reflects them from its surface so that they eventually all emerge parallel.

Internal reflection: Internal reflection occurs when the angle of incidence of a ray as it strikes an interface between two media is such that instead of being transmitted it is reflected. This happens at angles of incidence above a certain critical level. Internal reflection in quartz is used to cause ultraviolet light to pass down a specially cut quartz rod and be emitted only from the ends (Fig. 10.4).

2. Refraction: Refraction occurs when electromagnetic rays are transmitted from one medium to another with an angle of incidence greater than zero (Fig. 10.5).

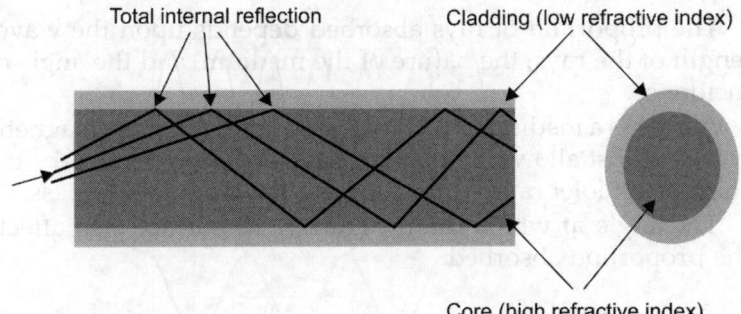

Fig. 10.4: Total internal reflection in quartz

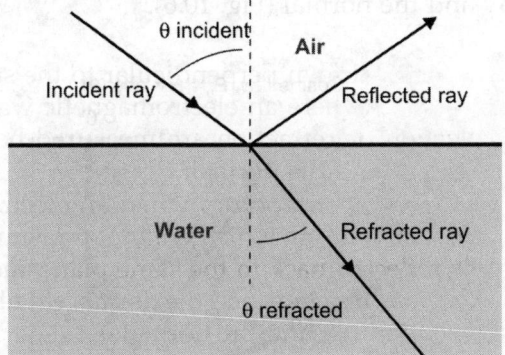

Fig. 10.5: Refraction of electromagnetic rays

Refraction causes the ray to be deflected from its original course by an amount depending on the media involved and the angle of incidence *(Snell's law)*.

When passing into an optically denser medium the ray is refracted towards the normal. When passing into a less dense medium, it is refracted away from the normal.

Absorption: When electromagnetic rays strike a new medium they may be absorbed and thus produce an effect.

Law of Grothus

The *law of Grothus* states that the rays must be absorbed on a surface to produce the effect.

The proportion of rays absorbed depends upon the wavelength of the rays, the nature of the medium, and the angle of incidence.

A filter is a medium which will absorb some electromagnetic waves whilst allowing others to pass. Cellophane absorbs the short ultraviolet rays while allowing the long ones to pass.

The angle at which the rays strike the surface also affects the proportion absorbed.

Lambert's Cosine Law

The *Lambert's cosine law* states that the intensity of the rays at the surface varies with the cosine of the angle between the incident ray and the normal (Fig. 10.6).

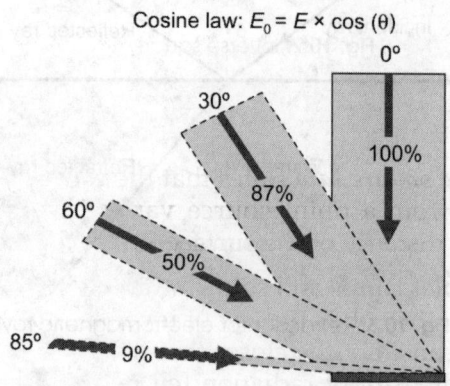

Cosine law: $E_0 = E \times \cos(\theta)$

Fig. 10.6: Lambert's cosine law

As cosine of $0° = 1$, to have maximum effect the radiation must be made to strike the surface at $90°$.

While applying ultraviolet and infrared lamps, ensure that the maximum number of rays strike the surface at $90°$ for the most effective treatment.

Inverse Square Law

The amount of rays absorbed is dependent upon the distance of the source from the surface (Fig. 10.7).

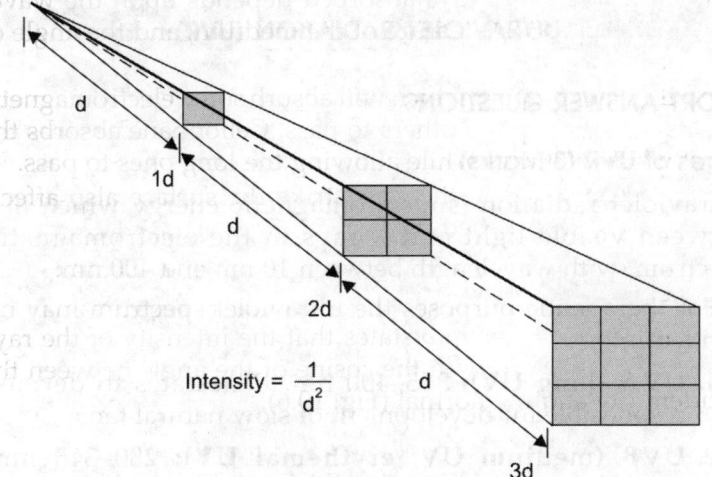

Fig. 10.7: Inverse square law

The *inverse square law* states that the intensity of radiation at a surface from a point source varies inversely with the square of the distance of the surface from that point source.

As ultraviolet lamps and some infrared lamps act almost as point sources, they obey the law of inverse square. In practical terms this means that the closer the patient to the source, the greater the intensity of radiation felt by the patient and vice versa.

Arndt-Schultz Law

The effect on body tissues is dependent on the amount of energy absorbed by the tissues.

Arndt-Schultz law states that no reaction or change will occur in the body tissues if the amount of energy absorbed is insufficient to stimulate the absorbing tissues.

According to this law, a certain minimum intensity of electromagnetic radiation is needed to initiate a biological process. Beyond a certain level, stronger intensity will have a progressively less positive effect and become inhibitory.

ULTRAVIOLET RADIATION (UVR)

SHORT ANSWER QUESTIONS

Types of UVR (3 Marks)

Ultraviolet radiation is electromagnetic energy which lies between visible light and X-rays in the electromagnetic spectrum, with wavelength between 10 nm and 400 nm.

For therapeutic purposes the ultraviolet spectrum may be divided into:

1. **UVA (long UV):** 315–400 nm. Penetrates to dermis, responsible for development of slow natural tan.
2. **UVB (medium UV, erythemal UV):** 280–315 nm. Produces new pigment formation, sunburn, vitamin D synthesis, responsible for inducing skin cancer.
3. **UVC (short UV, germicidal UV):** 100–280 nm. Does not reach the surface of the earth.

Tridymite Formation (3 Marks)

- The heat produced inside the burner or quartz tube causes some of it to change to another form of silica called tridymite.
- Tridymite is opaque to UVR. So, the total output of the lamp tends to fall as the proportion of tridymite increases.
- A variable resistance is included in the burner circuit to increase the potential difference across the burner and intensity of the current. Thus, the production of ultraviolet is increased but as less is transmitted by the quartz, output of the lamp is kept constant.

Types of UVR Generators (7 Marks)

1. High pressure mercury vapor lamp—air-cooled.
2. High pressure mercury vapor lamp—water-cooled (Kromayer lamp).
3. Fluorescent lamps

The UV apparatus is grouped as follows:

1. **Air-cooled lamps:** *Hanovia Alpine sun lamp* (Fig. 10.8) [high pressure vapor lamps], wavelength 253 nm (short wavelength) used in treatment of generalized skin conditions as acne and psoriasis.
   - Emit ultraviolet, infrared, and visible light. UVR produced falls within UV B range.
   - Mainly used to produce erythema and accompanying photochemical reactions.

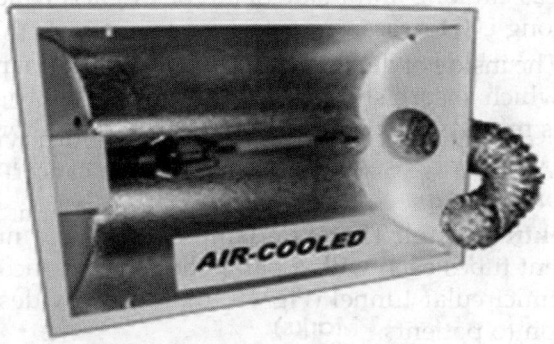

Fig. 10.8: Alpine sun lamp

2. **Water-cooled lamps:** *Kromayer lamp* (Fig. 10.9), wavelength at 366 nm give both UVA and UVB, used for treating localized lesions as pressure areas, ulcers, and sinuses in open areas.

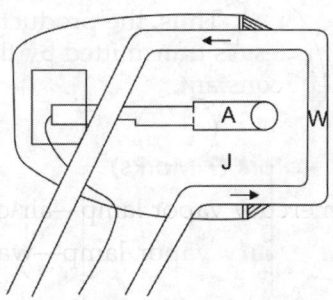

Fig. 10.9: Kromayer lamp

- Eliminates the danger of an IRR burn. The distilled water is circulated in the jacket in front of the Kromayer head. The purpose of which is to absorb the IRR.
- After the use of the lamp, the water circulation should be continued for 5 minutes after the burner is switched off in order to cool the lamp.

3. Fluorescent tubes

- The modern treatment methods often require the use of long UV without short UV. So, to meet these criteria the fluorescent tubes are used. Each tube is about 120 cm long and made of a type of glass which allows long UV to pass.
- The inside of the tube is coated with a special phosphor which absorb short UV. The output proportion of this is mainly of long UV, few IRR and some short UV.
- It is mainly used for general irradiation for individual or in group.

Theraktin tunnel: Theraktin lamp consists of a number of fluorescent tubes each with a parabolic reflector incorporated into a semicircular tunnel (Fig. 10.10). This provides an even irradiation to patients.

- Normally fluorescent tubes with a spectrum between 280 and 400 nm (UVA long) are used for treating large areas. It allows treatment of the whole body in 2 halves.
- All of the lamps should be positioned at least 18 inches from the patient.

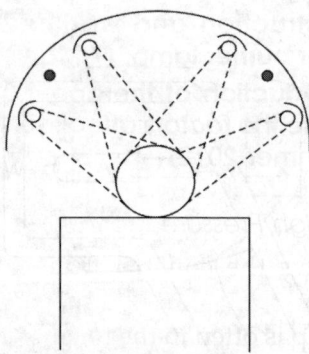

Fig. 10.10: Theraktin tunnel

Construction of Kromayer Lamp (7 Marks)

The Kromayer lamp is a water-cooled mercury vapor lamp, which eliminate the danger of an infrared burn (Fig. 10.9).

Construction

- The Kromayer lamp consists of a high pressure mercury vapor burner, the working of which is similar as for the air-cooled lamp. However, it is completely enclosed in a jacket of circulating distilled water, the purpose of which is to absorb the infrared.
- The burner is made up of quartz tube which allows the passage of ultraviolet.
- Enclosed in the tube is argon gas at low pressure. A small quantity of mercury is also enclosed in the tube and an electrode is sealed into either end.
- At the front of the Kromayer head the water circulates between two quartz windows which allow the ultraviolet to emerge. The water circulation should be continued for five minutes after the burner is switched off in order to cool the lamp.
- If a sinus is to be treated an applicator of quartz is fixed to the Kromayer head via a special attachment. These applicators convey the ultraviolet rays to their tip by total internal reflection.

LONG ANSWER QUESTIONS

1. **Describe construction and working of high pressure mercury vapour burner lamp. (7 Marks) (Summer 2017)**
2. **Explain the production of therapeutic air-cooled ultraviolet lamp. Write the factors affecting output of the lamp. (15 Marks) (Summer 2012)**

Construction of High Pressure Mercury Vapor Burner

Figure 10.11 shows the construction of a mercury vapor burner.

- The UVR lamp is often in the form of a U-shaped tube, so that it acts more or less as a point source of radiation.

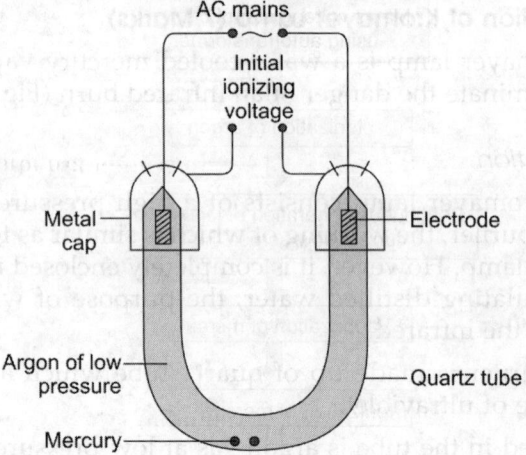

Fig. 10.11: Construction of a mercury vapor burner

- The burner is made up of quartz; this material allows the passage of ultraviolet and can withstand very high temperatures.
- The tube contains a small amount of argon gas at low, medium or high pressure.
- A small quantity of mercury is also enclosed in the tube.
- An electrode is sealed into either end and surrounding the ends are two metal caps across which a high potential difference is applied by incorporating an autotransformer into the circuit.

Production of Ultraviolet Radiation (Fig. 10.12)

- A high voltage is applied to the metal caps at either end, for a fraction of a second; by means of a separate step-up autotransformer into the circuit. In practice this is accomplished by pressing the 'start' button on the control panel, the mains voltage is step-up to 400 V which causes ionization of the argon atoms.
- Once the argon ionizes, normal mains voltage between the electrodes causes the positive and negative particles to move through the burner, so constituting an electric current.

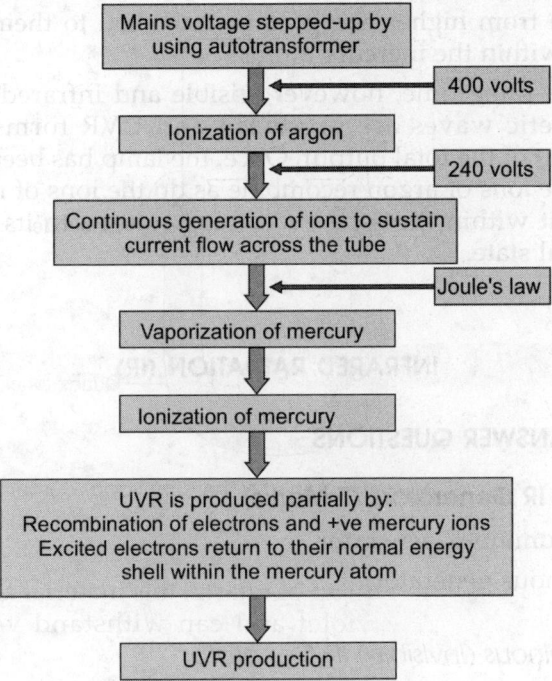

Fig. 10.12: Production of UVR

The electron move towards the positive terminal and then around the circuit, the positive ions move to the negative terminal and collect an electron. Overall, exactly the same number of electrons leaves the burner at the positive terminal as enter at the negative.

- As the two-way movement of the charged particles takes place, collision between moving ions and neutral argon atoms cause further ionization so that there is continuous generation of ionized particles to sustain the current flow across the tube. This flow of current across the tube generates heat (Joule's law), which eventually vaporizes the small amount of liquid mercury inside the tube and this mercury vapor itself becomes ionized.

- Ultraviolet radiation is produced partly as energy released by the recombination of electrons and the positive mercury ions, and partly by photons released when excited electrons return from higher energy quantum shell to their normal shell within the mercury atoms.

- At the same time, however, visible and infrared electromagnetic waves are produced and UVR forms only a portion of the total output. Once, the lamp has been turned off, the ions of argon recombine as do the ions of mercury, so that within the tube everything returns to its original neutral state.

INFRARED RADIATION (IR)

SHORT ANSWER QUESTIONS

Types of IR Generators (7 Marks)

1. Non-luminous generator
2. Luminous generator

Non-luminous (Invisible) IR Generator

A coil of wire wound on a cylinder of some insulating material such as fireclay or porcelain.

Construction

Parts of a non-luminous IR lamp

1. The emitter
2. The metal plate
3. Protective wire mesh
4. Parabolic reflector
5. Adjustable metal stand with screws
6. Base/wheel.
   - Usually the coil of wire is embedded in the fireclay, then the emission of rays (IR) is entirely from the fireclay which is commonly painted black. It is placed at the focal point of a parabolic reflector. This set-up is mainly to reflect the radiations into an approximately uniform beam.

- The parabolic reflector and emitter are mounted on a stand, firmly supported metal stand which can be adjusted to alter the height and angle of the reflector/ emitter.
- When such lamps are switched ON, they require some time to warm-up because of the thermal inertia of the considerable mass of metal and insulating material that has to be heated. The smaller lamp may take about 5 minutes and larger ones up to 15 minutes to reach maximum emission.

Luminous (Visible) IR Generator

- Luminous generators are produced by one or more incandescent lamps. Incandescent lamp consists of a tungsten filament in a large envelop which contains inert gas at low pressure. The inside part of the glass bulb is often silvered to provide reflector.
- This lamp work on the same principle as a simple electric bulb. On passing electric current, it gives off a continuous spectrum in the infrared and visible region and a few UVR.
- The radiation extends from the long infrared through the visible to the UVR. Some visible and UVR are absorbed by the reddened glass and are not transmitted by the lamp, whereas it gives a red visible emission.

Production of Non-luminous IR (7 Marks)

Principle of Production of Non-luminous IR

Joule's law: The Joule's law state that the amount of heat produced in a conductor is proportional to the square of the current (I^2), the resistance (R), and the time (t) for which the current flows through the circuit. This may be expressed as:

$Q = I^2Rt$

Where I = Current in amperes

R = Resistance in ohms

t = Time in seconds

Production: Any heated material will produce infrared radiations, the wavelength being determined by the temperature. Higher the temperature of the body the higher the mean frequency output consequently, the shorter the wave-length.

Infrared irradiation is produced as a result of molecular motion within heated materials. An increase in temperature above absolute zero results in the vibration or rotation of molecules within matter, which leads to the emission of infrared irradiation. Most convenient method to produce infrared is to heat a suitable resistance wire such as nickel-chrome alloy wound on a ceramic insulator.

Electric current → passed through the wires → produces heat.

IRs are emitted from the hot wires and from the fireclay which is heated by conduction.

Production of Luminous IR Lamp (Summer 2017) (7 Marks)

Principle of Production of Luminous IR

Spontaneous emission: Electron initially in level 2 "falls" to level 1 and gives off energy (just happens spontaneously) and energy is emitted in the form of a photon (Fig. 10.13).

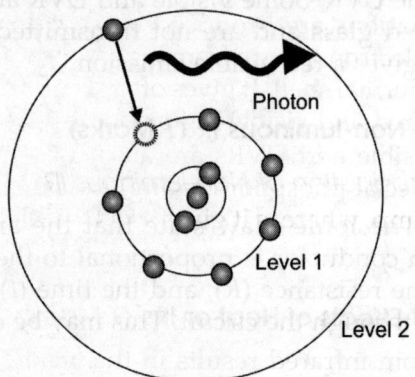

Fig. 10.13: Spontaneous emission

Construction

Luminous IRs are produced by one or more incandescent lamps. Incandescent lamp consists of a tungsten filament in a large envelop which contains inert gas at low pressure. The inside part of the glass bulb is often silvered to provide reflector (Fig. 10.14).

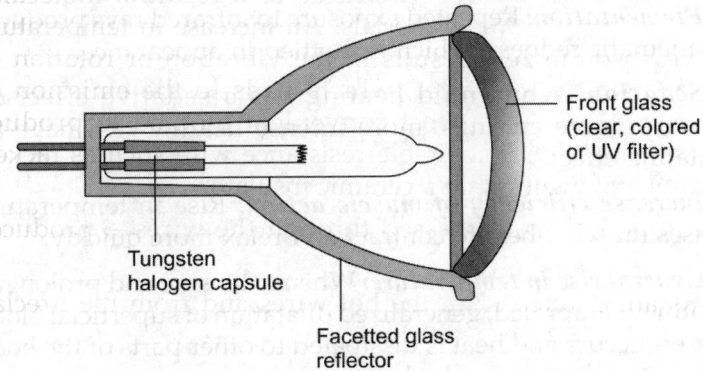

Fig. 10.14: Construction of luminous IR generator

Production

- This lamp works on the same principle as a simple electric bulb. On passing electric current, tungsten filament get heated (Joule's law), which causes excitation of electrons in the atoms of inert gas.
- The radiations are produced by photon released when excited electrons return from higher energy quantum shell to their normal shell. It gives off a continuous spectrum in the infrared and visible region and a few UVR.
- Some visible and UVRs are absorbed by the reddened glass (special phosphor coating) and are not transmitted by the lamp, whereas it gives a red visible emission along with IRs.

Physiological Effects of Heat or IRs (7 Marks)

Irradiation from infrared results in the production of heat in the superficial tissues and the heat is carried to the deeper tissues by conduction and by the circulating fluids. Physiological effects produced by IR are as follows:

Increased metabolism: It results in increased demands to oxygen and foodstuffs and increased output of waste products.

Vasodilatation: There is dilatation of capillaries and arterioles as the superficial sensory nerve endings causes reflex vasodilatation.

Pigmentation: Repeated exposure to infrared rays produces erythematic redness, which is mottled in appearance.

Sedation: While mild heating has a sedative effect on sensory nerve endings, more intense heating will have an irritating effect.

Increase efficiency of muscle action: Rise in temperature causes muscle fibers to contract and relax more quickly.

General rise in temperature: When extensive and prolonged treatment is applied, generalized dilatation of superficial blood vessels occurs and heat is dissipated to other parts of the body causing general rise in body temperature.

Fall in blood pressure: Generalized vasodilatation reduces peripheral resistance and blood viscosity, which tend to reduce blood pressure.

Increased activity of the sweat glands: The heated blood circulates throughout the body, affecting the centers concerned with regulation of temperature, which leads to increasing the activity of sweat glands.

Contraindications of IRs (7 Marks)

Contraindications of IRs are as follows

Impaired sensation: Patient will not be able to determine if the excessive heat is occurring.

Impaired circulation (atherosclerosis, DVT, Burger's disease): Unable to dissipate heat to other parts of the body, will lead to burns.

Dermatological conditions: Fungus, dermatitis and eczema may exacerbate.

Analgesic and narcotic drugs: It will raise the pain/thermal sensation threshold.

Deep X-ray therapy: Past 3 months, it reduces sensory appreciation.

Superficial metal implant: It retains the heat and will lead to a burn.

Eyes: The IRs can cause cataract.

Age: Elderly patients generally have impairment of sensation and circulation (lack of normal CVS response to heat may lessen the tolerance of thermal stress).

Acute infection: It will increase the infection processes.

Severe cardiac conditions: Heating a large area will cause an increase in cardiac output and the same may not be tolerated with severe cardiac patients.

Differences between Luminous and Non-luminous IRs (7 Marks)

Differences between luminous and non-luminous IRs are as follows:

Differences	Luminous IR	Non-luminous IR
Construction IR generators	Luminous IRs are produced by incandescent lamps. It consists of a tungsten filament in a large envelop which contains inert gas at low pressure.	A coil of resistance wire wound on a cylinder of some insulating materials. Electric current passes through wire and produces heat.
Heating time	Does not require heating time prior to treatment.	It takes about 5–15 minutes to be heated and emits their maximum intensity.
Wavelength	Ranges 350–4000 nm (maximum 1000 nm)	Ranges 1500–12000 nm (maximum 4000 nm)
Emission	Emits short IR (70%) and long IR (25%) along with visible light and ultraviolet rays.	Emits mostly long IR (>90%) and (10%) short IR and visible light.
Depth of penetration	Epidermis, dermis and subcutaneous tissue (5–10 mm)	Epidermis, and superficial dermis (1–2 mm)

(Contd.)

(Contd.)

Differences	Luminous IR	Non-luminous IR
Physiological effects	Pain reduction via counter-irritant effect.	Pain reduction via sedative effect.
Uses	Chronic inflammation	Acute inflammation
Treatment time	15–20 min	20–30 min
Distance from lamp	40–60 cm from treated area.	75–90 cm from treated area.

LASER

SHORT ANSWER QUESTIONS

Properties of Laser (3 Marks)

1. **Monochromaticity:** They are of single specific wavelength hence of defined frequency. In case of visible lasers, single specific color is produced, i.e. ruby laser gives red light at wavelength 694.3 nm (1 color–1 wavelength).
2. **Coherence:** They are in phase (Fig. 10.15).

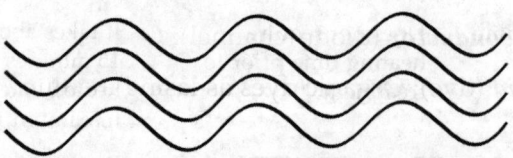

Fig. 10.15: Coherent light waves

Temporal coherence: Peak and troughs of both electric and magnetic fields occur at the same time.

Spatial coherence: They are all travelling in the same direction.

The distance over which the wavelengths stay in phase are called the *coherence length.*

3. **Collimation:** Lasers remain in a parallel beam. They do not diverge therefore the energy propagated over very long distances.

Differences between Ordinary Light and Laser Beam (3 Marks)

Differences between ordinary light and laser beam are as follows.

Ordinary light	Laser beam
Many different wavelengths	Monochromatic, i.e. single wavelength, one color
Multidirectional waves	Unidirectional waves
Incoherent waves	Coherent waves

Types of Laser (Summer 2012) (3 Marks)

Types of laser based on lasing medium are

- *Solid* crystal and glass (rod): Synthetic ruby
- *Gas* (chamber): He–Ne, argon, CO_2
- *Semiconductor* (diode–channel): Gallium arsenide
- *Liquid* (dye): Organic dyes as lasing medium.

Types of Laser Generators (7 Marks)

Ruby Laser (3 Marks)

Ruby laser consists of a small synthetic ruby rod made up of aluminum oxide. A helical xenon flash tube wound around it, gives an intense flash of white light. Both ends of the rod are made flat and silvered, one end being totally reflecting and the other partially transparent so that some radiations can be emitted. Wavelength of ruby laser is 694.3 nm (red light) (Fig. 10.16).

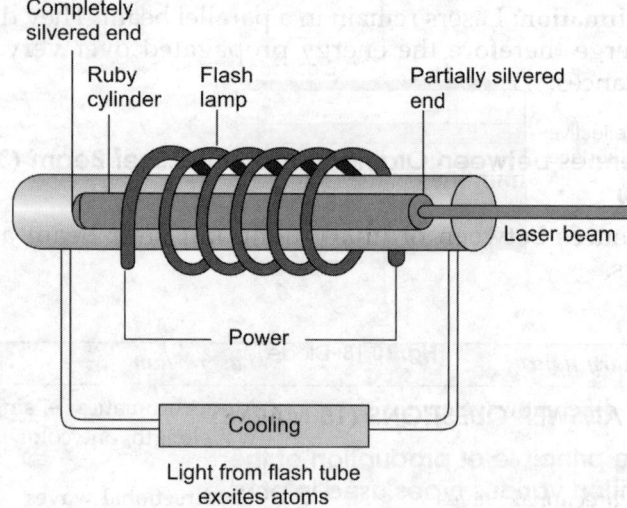

Fig. 10.16: Ruby laser

Helium–Neon Laser (3 Marks)

He–Ne stands for helium–neon. The He–Ne laser consists of a long tube containing helium and neon gas mixture at low pressure surrounded by flash gun tube. Wavelength of He–Ne laser is 632.8 nm (red light) (Fig. 10.17).

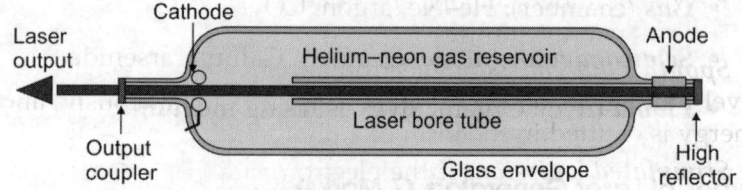

Fig. 10.17: He–Ne laser

Diode Laser (3 Marks)

These are specialized light-emitting diodes, based on semiconductor *p-n* junctions. They are of various kinds involving gallium, aluminum and arsenide (GaAlAs).

A diode laser produces an infrared (invisible) laser with wavelength between 904 and 910 nm (Fig. 10.18).

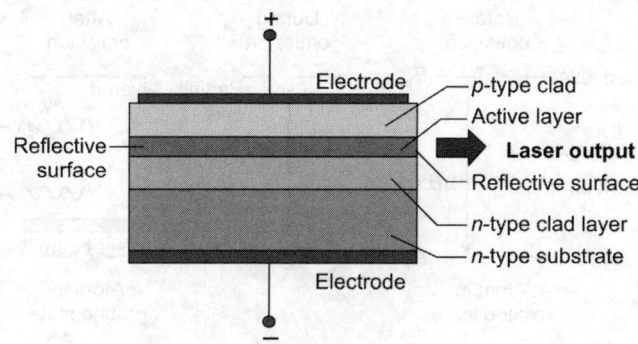

Fig. 10.18: Diode laser

LONG ANSWER QUESTIONS (15 MARKS)

1. Write principle of production of therapeutic laser.
2. Mention various types used in physiotherapy.
3. Explain production of laser beam. (15 Marks)

Principle of Production of Laser

The basic principle of production of the laser is spontaneous emission, absorption and stimulated emission of light.

Energy is quantized

- To raise an electron from one energy level to another, "input" energy is required.
- When falling from one energy level to another, there will be an energy "output".

Spontaneous emission: Electron initially in level 2 "falls" to level 1 and gives off energy (just happens spontaneously) and energy is emitted in the form of a photon (*refer* to Fig. 10.13).

Stimulated emission: If the electron is already in a higher energy state and can move to a lower level with a difference that corresponds to the energy of the stimulating photon. It may do so by giving out a photon of its own identical to that of the colliding photon. This process is called stimulated emission (Fig. 10.19).

Stimulated emission is the basis of production of laser and to achieve this two things are required.

1. Population inversion
2. Metastable state

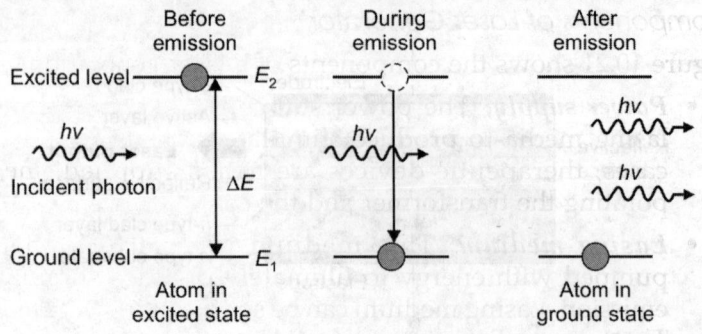

$$E_2 - E_1 = \Delta E = hv$$

Fig. 10.19: Stimulated emission

Population inversion: It needs many more atoms in the excited state than the ground state. This is called population inversion. Normally, more atoms are in the ground state than the excited state.

To achieve population inversion we must have metastable states and this is achieved by pumping.

Metastable states: These are excited states where electrons stay for unusually longer time. Normally, an electron in an excited state makes the transition to a lower state in a time of 10^{-7} sec. In contrast, an electron may stay in a metastable state for 10^{-3} sec (Fig. 10.20).

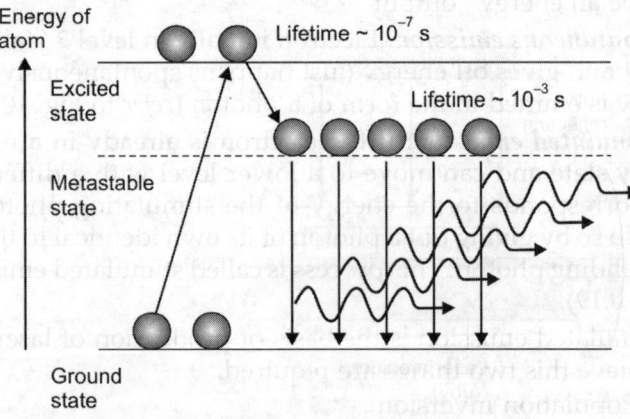

Fig. 10.20: Metastable state

Components of Laser Generator

Figure 10.21 shows the components of a laser generation.

- *Power supply:* The power source is used to pump the lasing media to produce stimulated emission. In most cases, therapeutic devices are mains supplied, incorporating the transformer and the control unit.

- *Lasing medium:* This medium is capable of being pumped with energy to ultimately produce stimulated emission. Lasing medium can be solid, liquid, or gaseous. The two media most commonly used are, the gaseous mixture of helium and neon (He–Ne) operating at a wavelength of 632.8 nm (i.e. red light) or gallium arsenide (Ga–As)/gallium–aluminum–arsenide (Ga–Al–As) semi-conductors typically producing radiations at 630–950 nm (visible red to near infrared).

- *Optical resonant cavity:* This is a chamber that contains lasing medium and incorporates a pair of parallel reflecting surfaces or mirrors. One mirror is fully reflecting, whereas another one is semitransparent mirror and so does not reflect 100% of light striking its surface. Within the chamber the photon of light produced by the lasing medium are reflected back and forth between the mirrors to ultimately produce an intense photon resonance.

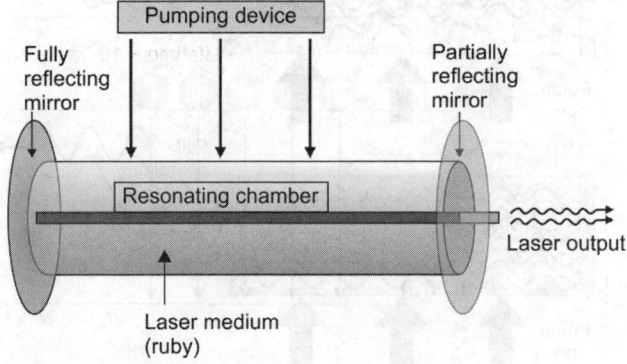

Fig. 10.21: Components of a laser generator

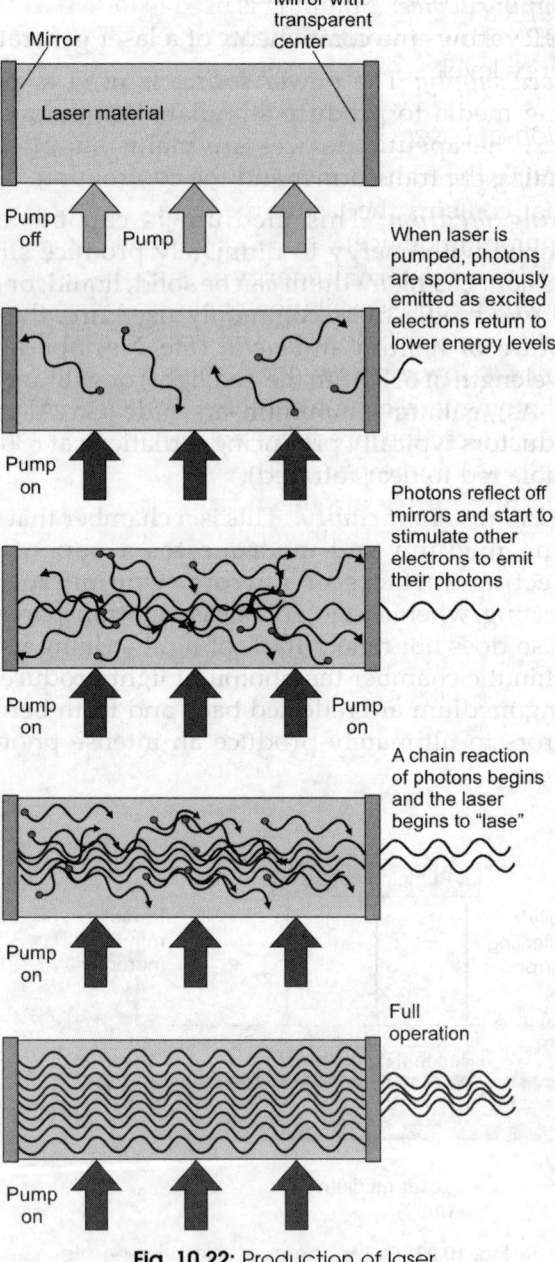

Fig. 10.22: Production of laser

- *Pumping device:* Pumping is used to describe the process of elevating an orbiting electron to a higher, excited energy level.

Production of Laser

Functional laser production requires 3 things: Optical resonant cavity that contains the lasing medium and external energy source (pumping device).

Electricity or external energy is supplied to the lasing medium which causes excitation of electrons to higher energy levels to attain metastable state. The electrons in the metastable state, jumps to lower energy level, releasing a photon.

The photon interacts with another electron in the metastable state. This interaction produces another photon at the same wavelength and same phase. These photons are reflected by fully reflecting mirror at one end and the laser light is then emitted through the partially reflective mirror at the other end (Fig. 10.22).

Superficial Heating Modalities

PARAFFIN WAX BATH

Methods of Application of Paraffin Wax Bath (7 Marks) (Summer 2017)

Paraffin wax bath therapy is an application of molten paraffin wax over the body parts. Paraffin wax therapy provides about six times the amount of heat available in water because the mineral oil in the paraffin lowers its melting point.

Knobs

It consists of stainless steel container, mains, thermostat, pilot lamp, power pilot lamp, lid and caster (Fig. 11.1).

Power knob: It is used to control the power of the machine.

Temperature control: It is used to regulate temperature of the wax. It is regulated by thermostat.

Pilot lamp (red): It glows when the wax is heated

Pilot lamp (green): It glows when the machine is on.

Lid: It is used to cover the wax bath.

Caster: Used to move the apparatus from one place to another.

Outer and inner jacket: To preserve the heat of the molten wax.

Preparation of Apparatus

The machine is switched on 30–45 minutes prior to the treatment to melt the wax.

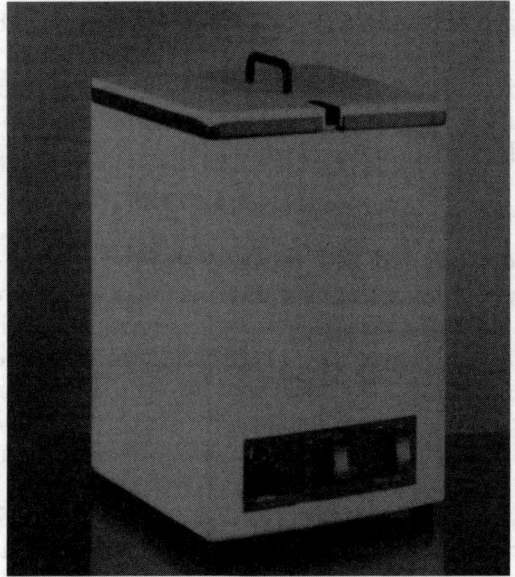

Fig.11.1: Paraffin wax bath unit

The thermostat is fixed to maintain the temperature between 42°–52°C. The red pilot indicates that the wax has melted.

The wax bath has paraffin oil/mineral oil (7:1) added to it as impurity as these added impurity help to produce a temperature between 42° and 52°C with an adequate lubricating effect, which helps in supplying and easy removal from the body.

Preparation of Patient

The patient is given a comfortable position according to the joint to be treated. The part to be treated is exposed with the prior permission of the patient.

The nature of wax treatment is explained and the area to be treated is inspected for contraindication like open wound, skin infection, ischemic condition, skin allergy and the most important for defective skin sensation.

This includes the testing of sensitivity of skin to heat and cold which is done by taking 2 test tubes, one containing warm water at 40°–45°C and other containing cold water at 10°–15°C.

The tubes are applied randomly to the body part to be treated, to find out the sensitivity to heat and cold.

The part to be treated is washed with water and makes it dry thoroughly to prevent water from entering the wax bath. Any jewellery from the part should be removed.

METHODS OF APPLICATION

1. **Dip and wrap:** In this method the part to be treated is immersed in wax bath for 1–2 seconds and removed and allowed to cool for 2–3 seconds. It is reimmersed in the bath for about 6–12 times till a layer of 2–3 mm thickness of wax is formed evenly. The part is then wrapped in plastic bag and then by a Turkish towel to prevent heat loss to the environment. If there is provocation of edema, the part should be kept elevated. The part is then left for 15–20 minutes. After 15–20 minutes of solidification of the wax by which time it has turned into a glove of wax, the wax is removed and put inside the tank for reuse (Fig. 11.2).

2. **Brushing method:** If the part cannot be dipped inside the bath, it is possible to coat the surface by painting with the use of a large brush. It is commonly used for areas like the hip, knee, elbow, shoulder, etc. After 2–3 mm thickness of wax is painted, the part is covered by a plastic sheet to prevent

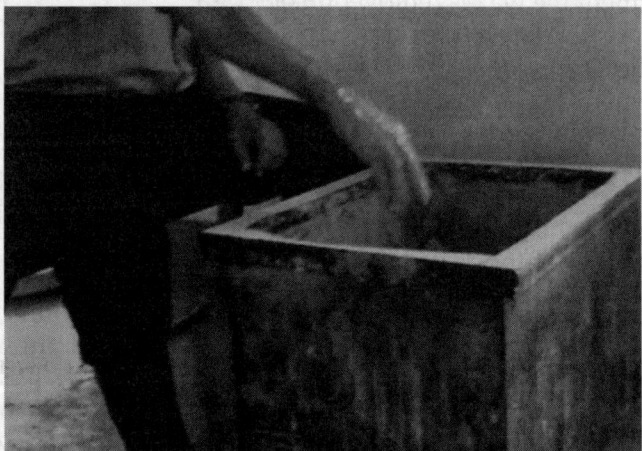

Fig. 11.2: Wax therapy to hand by dipping method

heat loss. After solidification (15 minutes later) the wax glove is removed into the tank for re-use.

3. **Pouring method:** For areas like the knee, elbow where the dipping is not possible, another alternative method is pouring. In this method, the part to be treated is positioned over a large bowl and using a shallow spoon with insulated handle molten wax is poured over the body part. After 2–3 mm of wax is built over the part it is covered with a plastic sheet to prevent heat loss. The treatment is terminated after 15 minutes by removing the wax layer from the body into the tank for re-use.

4. **Bandaging method:** In this method, bandages of a suitable size and mesh are soaked in hot molten wax and then wrapped around the body part. Additional wax can also be brushed over the bandage. After wrapping, the part is covered by a plastic sheet. After 15 minutes, the bandages of wax are removed and the wax is separated into the tank. This method is suitable for areas like the back, shoulder, hip, etc.

Termination

The procedure is carried out for 15–20 minutes and the patient is instructed not to move as it may crack the layer of wax and prevent equal distribution of heat. After the end of the treatment the wax is removed in one piece without any breaks. The area is checked for redness, swelling.

The wax is put back into the bath and then purified. After treatment the area around the wax bath unit is cleaned as it may be dangerous to the patient as well as the therapist (chance of falling due to slippery floor).

Describe the physiological effects of superficial heat. Write down the methods of application of paraffin wax bath. (7 + 8 = 15 Marks)

OR

Explain physiological effects of heat. Describe in detail paraffin wax bath along with indications and contraindications. (15 Marks)

OR

Write principle of paraffin wax therapy. Describe methods of applications and physiological effects of PWB therapy. (15 Marks)

Physiological effects of superficial heat are as follows

1. *Increased metabolism:* This is in accordance with van't Hoff's law, which states that any chemical change capable of being accelerated is accelerated by rise in temperature. The increase in metabolism is greatest in region where most heat is produced, i.e. in superficial tissue. As a result of increased metabolism there is as increased demand for oxygen and foodstuffs, and an increase output of waste products, including metabolites.

2. *Vasodilatation:* There is dilatation of the capillaries and arterioles in the superficial tissues. This is due to the direct effect of the heat on the blood vessels, causing vasodilatation. The action of the metabolites on the walls of the capillaries and arterioles causing dilatation of these vessels and, unless the heating is very mild to irritation of the superficial sensory nerve endings, can also cause a reflex dilatation of the arterioles. Thus, the flow of blood to the superficial tissues is increased, and increased supply of oxygen and foodstuffs is made available, and waste products are removed.

3. *Pigmentation:* Following repeated exposure to infrared rays there may be an increase in pigmentation. The erythema produced by superficial heat appears as soon as the part become warm and begins to fade soon after the exposure of heat ceases. It is mottled in appearance and may be observed in the legs of individuals who habitually sit close to the fire. The pigmentation arises in a different way from that which follows ultraviolet irradiation, due to the destruction of red blood cells.

4. *Effects on sensory nerves:* Mild heating appears to have a sedative effect on the sensory nerve endings, while more intense heating has an irritating effect. The irritating effect is more marked in irradiation with the luminous than with the non-luminous generator, but this is probably due to the action of the shorter visible and ultraviolet rays rather than to that of the infrared rays.

5. *Effects on muscle tissue:* Rise in temperature induces muscle relaxation and increases the efficiency of muscle action, as the increased blood supply ensures the efficiency of muscle contraction, the fibers contract and relaxes more quickly and relaxation of the antagonists permits a freer action of the prime muscles.

6. *General rise in temperature:* This occurs if the treatments are extensive and prolonged. The blood in the superficial vessels is heated, and then passes to other parts of the body, causing a general rise in temperature. In association with this there may be a generalized dilatation of the superficial blood vessels, due to the effect of the heated blood on the centers concerned with regulation of body temperature.

7. *Fall in blood pressure:* If there is generalized vasodilatation the peripheral resistance is reduced, and this causes a fall in blood pressure. Heat reduces the viscosity of the blood, and this also tends to reduce the blood pressure.

8. *Increased activity of sweat glands:* There is reflex stimulation of the sweat glands in the area exposed to the heat, resulting from the effect of the heat on the sensory nerve endings. As the heated blood circulates throughout the body it affects the centers concerned with regulation of temperature, and there is increased activity of the sweat glands throughout the body. When this generalized sweating occurs there is increased elimination of waste products.

Indications of Paraffin Wax Bath (3 Marks)

Pain and muscle spasm: Wax reduces the pain and muscle spasm seen in hands and feet, as the moist heat encircles each finger and toe and relives pain.

Edema and inflammation: The gentle heat reduces post-traumatic swelling of the hands and feet, and also swelling in hands affected by rheumatoid arthritis or degenerative joint disease, particularly in the subacute and early chronic stages of inflammation.

Adhesions and scars: Wax softens the adhesions and scars in the skin and thus facilitates the mobilization and stretching procedures.

Contraindications of Paraffin Wax Bath (7 Marks)

Impaired skin sensation: Patient will not be able to determine if the excessive heat is occurring.

This will be determined by a hot/cold skin sensation test.

Circulatory dysfunction: Patients with varicose veins, deep vein thrombosis and arterial disease must not have any heat applied directly over the affected part.

Some dermatological conditions: Dermatological conditions such as eczema, athlete's foot and dermatitis may exacerbate by moist heat.

Infections and open wounds: Heat will increase the infective activity.

Cancer and tuberculosis: Heat increases the metabolic rate (van't Hoff's law) thereby increasing the rate of growth and spread the disease in the area to be treated.

Analgesic drugs: If the patients are taking strong narcotics for pain, heat is not administered immediately after intake of drugs, since pain tolerance to heat is impaired.

Deep X-ray therapy: Within three months prior to treatment decreased blood flow in the area and may cause impaired skin sensation.

Gross edema: With a very thin and delicate skin covering the area, the skin may be damaged and the heat may tend to increase the edema.

HYDROCOLLATOR PACK UNIT

Methods of Application of Hydrocollator Packs (7 Marks)

Hydrocollator packs are available commercially, such as those made from bentonite, a hydrophilic silicate gel covered with canvas. The packs are made up of different sizes for application to the different body parts. They are stored in water kept at about 75°–80°C, in a tank with electric heater controlled by thermostat (Fig. 11.3).

Knobs

Mains: It is used to indicate the machine is switched on/off.

Thermostat: It is used to regulate the temperature.

Control knob: It is used to control the power.

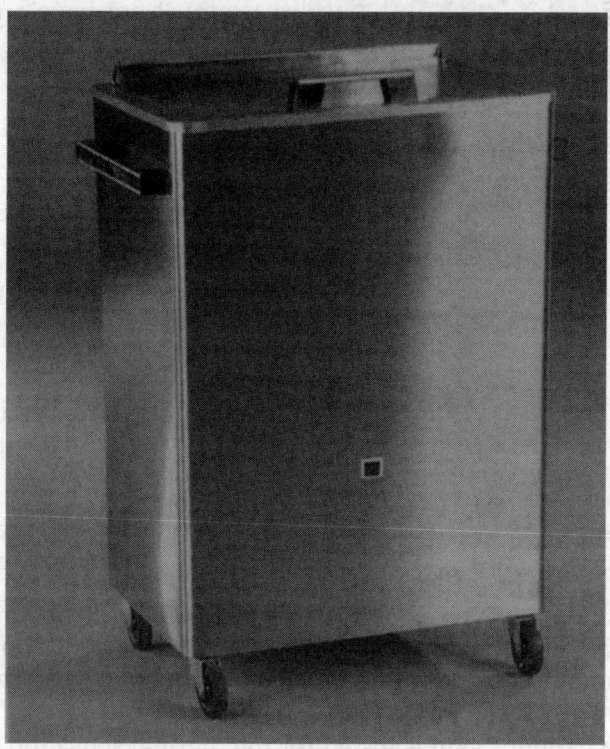

Fig. 11.3: Hydrocollator pack unit

Preparation of Apparatus

The hot pack is selected of particular size depending upon the area to be treated. The pack is kept inside the hydrocollator tank and it is allowed to be heated to a particular temperature.

The towel of particular size is folded in 4 to 8 layers which are required to maintain the temperature within 42°C, although the pack is kept at a temperature of about 75°C (Fig. 11.4).

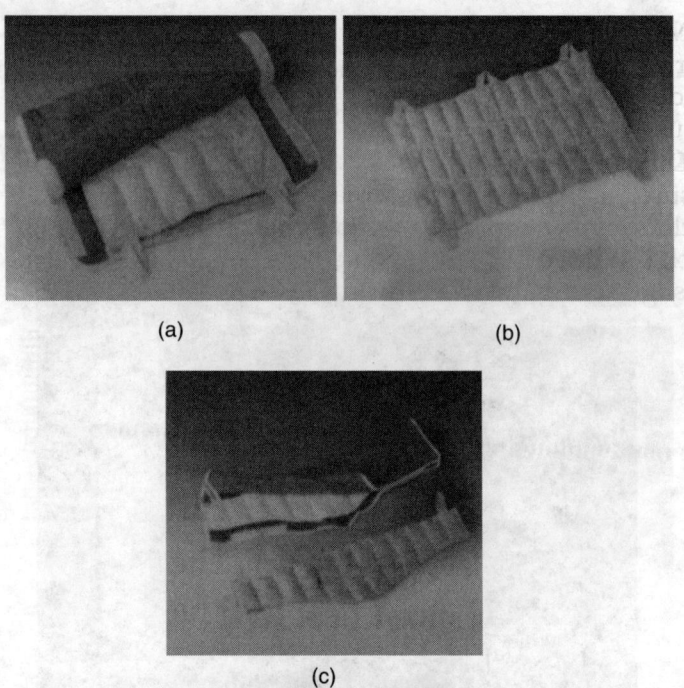

(a)   (b)

(c)

Fig. 11.4a to c: Hydrocollator hot packs

Preparation of Patient

The patient is given a comfortable position for the therapy and the part to be treated is undressed. The patient should be explained about the nature of the treatment. Any ornament presents over the part to be treated is removed.

The patient's skin is tested for the thermal sensation. Check for all the contraindications like open wounds, skin infections, impaired skin sensation, cancer, allergic rashes, etc.

Application Procedure

The gel pack is taken out from the unit by a tongue, remove excess water and place it on the towel. Fold another towel into 4–6 layers and place it over the pack. Wrap the whole pack up with the bottom towel. The temperature of the wrapped pack should not exceed the 44°C. The pack is placed over the part to be treated and kept in position for 20–30 minutes.

Monitor the initial response from the patient to treatment during the first 5 to 10 minutes by asking the patient for feedback and by visually inspecting the skin. If necessary, adjust the layers of toweling.

During the treatment maintain the position of hot pack and ensure that it does not exacerbate pain, produce discomfort or occlude circulation. After the treatment is over remove the hot pack and inspect the treatment area. It is normal for the area to be slightly red and to feel warm to touch (Fig. 11.5).

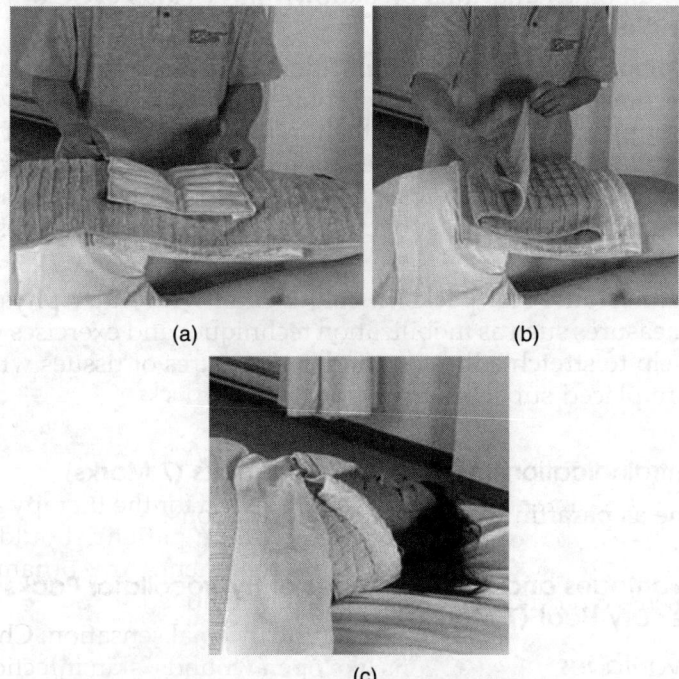

(a)   (b)

(c)

Fig. 11.5a to c: Application procedure of hydrocollator packs

Indications of Hydrocollator Packs (3 Marks)

- **Relief of pain:** Hydrocollator packs are widely used for the relief of pain. Most therapeutic heating is of the skin, this suggests that the major pain relieving effects are mainly reflex, possibly an activation of the pain gate mechanism. Pain is also possibly relieved by heat reducing the level of muscle spasm usually associated with it.

- **Reduction of muscle spasm:** Heat may reduce muscle spasm by reducing the level of ischemia associated with prolonged contraction in affected muscles. Increasing the muscle temperature to about 42°C results in inhibition of the motor neuron pool by increased firing from Golgi tendon organ and a reduced level of excitation by the muscle spindle due to reduced gamma efferent activity, thus reduces tone of the muscle. The rise in temperature also causes increased circulation which removes pain metabolites and thus breakdown the vicious cycle of pain and muscle spasm.

- **Edema and inflammation:** Edematous areas over a large section of an extremity, in chronic stages, can be treated with a hot pack in elevation of the limb to help absorption of the exudates. Temperature elevation of 2° to 5°C will cause an increase in phagocytosis and aid absorption of exudates, particularly in the subacute and early chronic stages of inflammation.

- **Adhesions:** Hot packs in conjunction with other physical measures such as mobilization techniques and exercises will help to stretch adhesions and contractures of tissues which are placed superficially.

Contraindications of Hydrocollator Packs (7 Marks)

Same as paraffin wax bath contraindications.

Advantages and Disadvantages of Hydrocollator Packs Over Dry Heat (7 Marks)

Advantages

1. A hydrocollator pack is easy to apply. They are of various sizes which fit most clinical needs.
2. The patient does not need much handling. The pads can be laid out ready for the patient to place on the affected part.
3. Moist heat has a more sedative effect than dry heat.
4. Low cost, minimal maintenance, long life.
5. Maximal temperatures are more uniform than in electrically-heated pads.

Disadvantages

1. A hydrocollator pack is not easily applied around shoulders and hips.
2. It is somewhat heavy and should not be used on extremely sensitive patients, since it can create discomfort.
3. Sometimes moist packs have a tendency to cause a skin rash.

CRYOTHERAPY

SHORT ANSWER QUESTIONS (3 MARKS)

1. Circulatory Response to Cooling (Nov-Dec 2009)

- Cold application causes reflex vasoconstriction of cutaneous vessels. Application of cold causes increase in sympathetic nerves activity, smooth muscle contraction and may increase viscosity of blood. All these changes result in reduced blood flow in the area that is directly cooled. However, when the temperature is reduced there is cold-induced vasodilatation may occur.
- Vasodilatation and vasoconstriction tend to occur in a cyclical manner. The repeated cyclical vasodilatation and vasoconstriction are known as hunting reaction.

2. Lewis Hunting Reaction (Winter 2010 and 2011)

- In 1930, Lewis stated that following the application of intense cold in the body there was a vasoconstriction with the liberation of histamine-like (H) substances produced by the intense cold and noxious stimuli.
- When there were sufficient 'H' substances, vasodilatation occurred for a brief period of time about 4 to 6 minutes and their vasodilatation removed all the 'H' substances.
- Vasoconstriction was established again, with vasodilatation occurring at farther interval. This apparent 'hunting' for a mean point of circulation is called Lewis's hunting reaction (Fig. 11.6).

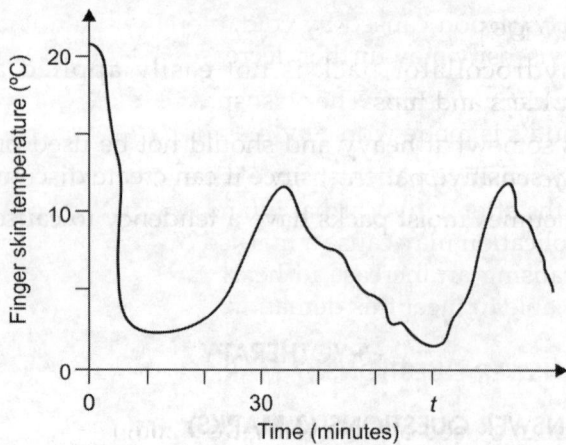

Fig. 11.6: Lewis's hunting reaction

3. Uses of Ice Therapy

OR

Three Indications of Cryotherapy (3 Marks)

1. *Muscle spasm:* Cryotherapy is effective in relieving the muscle spasm. Relief of spasm may occur due to decreased muscle spindle activity and secondary to the relief of pain.
2. *Pain relief:* Cold is one of the highly effective physio-therapeutic modalities in relieving pain. It is commonly used for the relief of acute pain. It can also be used for the relief of acute exacerbation of pain on the chronic back-ground, pain relief may occur due to counterirritation, reduced nerve conduction, decreased inflammatory process and relief of muscle spasm.
3. *Swelling:* Cold application can reduce the swelling following an acute injury. It may be due to vasoconstriction of arterioles and reduction in extravasations of fluid into interstitial space.

4. Contraindications of Cryotherapy (3 Marks)

Contraindications of cryotherapy are as follows

1. *Peripheral vascular disease:* In conditions such as arteriosclerosis, there is an impairment of circulation over a particular area which is contraindicated, as the immediate

vasoconstriction caused by cold, along with an increase of blood viscosity may further decreases the blood circulation.

2. *Vasospastic disease:* The vasospasm in diseases such as Raynaud's is made worse by the application of ice.

3. *Cardiac conditions:* Ice treatment should be avoided for 6 months after a myocardial infarct. The initial shock of the ice application may cause a marked drop in blood pressure, thus causing an increase in heart rate—a weak heart may not be able to meet this demand.

SHORT ANSWER QUESTIONS (7 MARKS)

1. Therapeutic uses of Cold (Nov-Dec 2009)

a. Acute inflammation

Cryotherapy is widely used to control acute inflammation and to accelerate recovery from injury.

- It decreases cellular metabolic rate thus helps to reduce secondary hypoxic injury.
- It gives symptomatic relief from the inflammatory response.
- It enhances function by decreasing pain by pain gate mechanism at spinal cord level.

It is recommended to apply cold immediately following an injury and throughout the acute inflammatory phase that lasts for 48–72 hours. The duration of treatment is limited to 15 minutes or less.

b. Pain relief: Cold is one of the highly effective physio-therapeutic modalities in relieving pain. It is commonly used for the relief of acute pain. It can also be used for the relief of acute exacerbation of pain on the chronic background.

Cryotherapy can decrease pain due to direct and indirect effects.

The direct effect is the modification of pain sensation (counterirritation) by pain gate mechanism. The indirect effect can be due to its interruption of the pain-spasm-pain cycle and alleviation of underlying cause of pain such as edema or inflammation.

c. **Muscle spasm:** Spasm is a normal response to injury or pain, and is manifested as an increase in muscle tone in a specific area with the apparent aim of limiting movement and further damage. However, the sustained contraction of muscle itself starts to produce pain, often resulting in spasm.

Cryotherapy is effective in relieving the muscle spasm. Relief of spasm may occur due to decreased muscle spindle activity, reduced velocity of nerve conduction, and secondary to relief of pain.

d. **Swelling/edema:** Cold application can reduce localized swelling following an acute injury. The alternate periods of vasoconstriction and vasodilatation affect the capillary blood flow, and it is across the capillary membrane that tissue fluid and metabolic exchanges take place. Consequently excess tissue fluid can be removed from the area and returned to the systemic circulation. Increased circulation allows more nutrients and repair substances into damaged areas. Thus, ice is very useful in removing swelling and aiding repair. For example, ice-cube massage may be used to accelerate the rate of repair of bedsores.

e. **Reduction of spasticity:** Cryotherapy has been found to reduce spasticity in patients with upper motor neuron disorders. Cold applied for longer periods (up to 30 min) reduces the conduction velocity of the motor nerve supplying the spastic muscle groups and depressed sensitivity of receptors such as the muscle spindle which can inhibit the contraction of spastic muscles causing reduction of spasticity.

f. **Facilitation of muscle contraction:** The excitatory stimulus of quick icing is used to facilitate contraction of muscles following regeneration of a mixed peripheral nerve or where muscles are inhibited postoperatively or to facilitate the antagonistic muscles of the spastic groups in upper motor neuron (UMN) lesion.

When cold is applied in an appropriate way the skin stimulus of ice can be used to increase the excitatory bias around the anterior horn cells. Combined with other forms of excitation and with the patient's volition, this can often produce contraction in an inhibited muscle.

g. An adjunctive measure for exercises and stretching (cryokinetic and cryostretch)

In cryokinetics: Cold is applied for 20 minutes or more to produce numbness, following which the patient exercises the part for 3–5 minutes or till the sensation returned.

In cryostretch: The cooling agent is applied before stretching to reduce spasm and pain thereby facilitating better stretching of the tight structures.

2. Methods of Cold Application (7 Marks)

Methods of application: 1. Ice towel, 2. Ice pack, 3. Immersion

1. Ice towel: A popular method of application because there is a little danger of producing ice burn.

Preparation: Prepare the bed by removing the blanket and sheets, and cover it with waterproof material.

Adequately expose the part to be treated; protecting any clothing that the patient needs to wear.

Prepare the ice solution by filling bucket or large bowl with two parts of flaked or crushed ice to one part water. This mix should give mulch, in which two terry towels are immersed.

Application: The surplus water is wrung from one towel, leaving as much ice clinging to it as possible. The towels are changed when they have been in position for at least 30 seconds, but not longer than 2 minutes.

Up to ten towels can be applied consecutively, more if the physiotherapist considers they will be beneficial, i.e. the total treatment time is of the order of 15–20 minutes.

2. Ice packs: Crushed or flaked ice is taken in a plastic bag large enough for the area to be treated which can be molded to body part.

Preparation of bed: A gutter made of polythene sheet is folded and placed on the bed. A folded towel is placed underneath its edges in order to channel the water produced from the melting ice into a container at the side of the bed. The gutter will be positioned below the part to be treated.

Preparation of patient: The part to be treated is exposed and put into a comfortable position over the prepared gutter. A vegetable or nut oil is spread over the skin on which the ice pack is to be placed. This is to try and prevent an ice burn.

Application: The wet ice pack is placed on top of the part to be treated. Pack should never surround a limb as this would inevitably put pressure on one aspect of the limb and could reduce the circulation locally. A reduced circulation would prevent a normal circulation response to cooling and might precipitate an ice burn. The pack may be left in position for between 10 and 20 minutes.

3. **Immersion:** It is a technique in which the part to be treated is immersed in ice solution, unfortunately it is only practical to immerse certain areas, such as hands, feet and elbows.

Preparation: The solution is made up of 50% ice and 50% water placed in a suitable container.

Application: The patient immerses the part in the solution and keeps it in either for a single ten minute session or for a series of shorter immersion until a cumulative total of 10 minutes has been reached. Often the patient experiences intense pain in the immersed area, sometimes severe enough to cause him to faint, he should therefore be suitably supported, and watched throughout the treatment.

3. Physiological Effect and uses of Ice Therapy (Winter 2012)

Physiological effects of cryotherapy are as follows:

a. **Reduced body temperature:** Cold causes fall in local body temperature. However, severe local cooling may result in hypothermia. Hypothermia is a condition where the core temperature is below 35°C. It may be a life-threatening situation.

b. **Circulatory effect:** Cold application causes reflex vaso-constriction of cutaneous vessels. Application of cold causes increase in sympathetic nerves activity, smooth muscle contraction and may increase viscosity of blood. All these changes result in reduced blood flow in the area that is directly cooled. However, when the temperature is reduced below 10°C then cold inducted reflex vasodilatation may occur. Reflex vasodilatation tends to occur in a cyclical manner and is believed to result from an axon reflex. Reflex vasodilatation following cold application was first reported by Lewis in 1930. The repeated cyclical vasodilatation and vasoconstriction are known as Lewis hunting response.

c. **Reduction in metabolism:** Cooling of tissue decreases the cellular metabolic rate and hence the energy and oxygen requirements of cells get reduced which help to prevent secondary hypoxic injury. That is why cold is selected in acute inflammation, where there is an abnormal increase in the demand for the metabolic activity.

d. **Decreases nerve conduction velocity:** The nerve conduction velocity decreases in proportion to the degree of cooling. Cold can decrease the velocity of conduction in both sensory as well as motor nerves and has a greater effect on myelinated and small diameter fibers ($A\delta$) than unmyelinated and large diameter fibers. Reversible total nerve conduction block also occurs, if ice is applied over the nerve trunk where it is superficial.

e. **Increase in pain threshold:** A decrease in pain after cold application occurs due to the increased pain threshold because of counterirritation via the pain gate mechanism and the reduction of muscle spasm and sensory nerve conduction velocity.

Stimulation of cutaneous cold receptors provides sufficient sensory stimulus which can block the transmission of painful stimuli, partially or fully, along the spinal cord to the sensory cortex, increasing pain threshold and decreasing pain sensation.

f. **Alteration of muscle strength:** The effect of cold on muscle strength is variable. It has been found that cold applied for 5 minutes or less causes an increase in muscle strength (isometric). The proposed mechanism for the increase in strength with short duration cold is that brief cooling causes increase of excitability of motor nerve.

When cold is applied for 30 minutes or longer causes a decrease of the muscle strength initially followed by an increase (isometric strength). After prolonged cooling the initial decrease of muscle strength is due to the fact that, there is a decrease in muscle blood flow, increase of muscle viscosity, reduction of motor nerve conductivity and increased joint stiffness. After the initial decrease of the muscle strength, the increase of strength could be due to increase blood flow and decrease viscosity of muscle brought about by cold-induced vasodilatation.

g. **Facilitation of muscle contraction:** Brief cold when applied to the muscle with intact lower motor neuron is found to facilitate the muscle contraction which could be due to enhance excitability of the alpha motor neuron to this brief cooling.

h. **Decrease of muscle spasticity:** Cryotherapy has been found to decrease spasticity for a temporary period which could be due to summated mechanism of decrease of gamma motor neuron activity, followed by decrease in afferent spindle and Golgi tendon organ activity.

It is usually recommended to apply ice for up to 30 minutes to cause a decrease of spasticity lasting for 1–1.5 hours. During this period therapeutic activities can be carried out.

4. Methods of Application of Ice in Cryotherapy (Summer 2012)

OR

Methods of Ice Application (Winter 2011)

Various methods of application of cryotherapy are as follows:

1. **Ice towel:** A popular method of application because there is a little danger of producing ice burn.

   Preparation: Prepare the bed by removing the blanket and sheets, and cover it with waterproof material.

   Adequately expose the part to be treated; protecting any clothing that the patient needs to wear.

   Prepare the ice solution by filling bucket or large bowl with two parts of flaked or crushed ice to one part water. This mix should give mulch, in which two terry towels are immersed.

Application: The surplus water is wrung from one towel, leaving as much ice clinging to it as possible which is then applied to the part being treated. The towels are changed when they have been in position for at least 30 seconds, but not longer than 2 minutes.

Up to ten towels can be applied consecutively, more if the physiotherapist considers they will be beneficial, i.e. the total treatment time is of 15–20 minutes.

Modification of technique

- In the presence of swelling:
  - It is permissible to elevate the limb and completely surround the joint with the ice towel.
  - Patient can exercise with the towel in position.
  - Therapist can apply manual resistance technique with the towel in position.
- When treating spastic muscles:
  - The towels are applied along the length of the muscle from origin to insertion.

2. **Ice-packs:** Crushed or flaked ice may be placed in terry towel folded into an appropriate shape. Indicated for acute injuries and prevention of swelling following exercise of injured area.

Preparation: A gutter made of polythene sheet is folded and placed on the bed. A folded towel is placed underneath its edges in order to channel the water produced from the melting ice into a container at the side of the bed. The gutter will be positioned below the part to be treated.

The part to be treated is exposed and put into a comfortable position over the prepared gutter.

A vegetable or nut oil is spread over the skin on which the ice-pack is to be placed. This is to try and prevent an ice burn.

Making an ice-pack: Spread out a terry towel on a flat surface. Arrange a one-inch thick layer of crushed-ice (enough to cover the treatment site) in the middle of the towel.

Fold the long edges of the towel to overlap one another and the ice. Roll up the ends of the towel toward one another to make handling easy. Before applying to the treatment site, moisten the side of the ice-pack that will touch the skin with water (Figs 11.7 and 11.8).

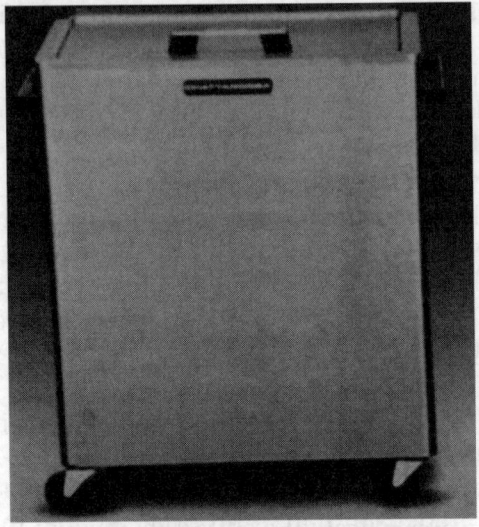

Fig. 11.7: Cold packs unit

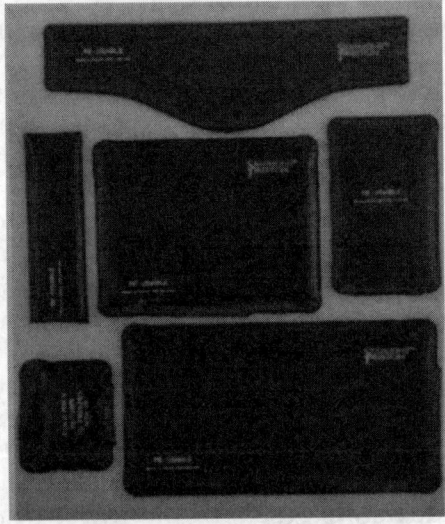

Fig. 11.8: Cold packs

Commercial cold packs

- An *ice bag* may be created by putting ice in a plastic bag or by freezing a moistened hydrocollator.
- Do not apply directly to skin.
- A *damp towel* should be wrapped around the ice bag to prevent any part of it from directly touching the unprotected skin.

Application: The wet ice pack is placed on top of the part to be treated. Pack should never surround a limb as this would inevitably put pressure on one aspect of the limb and could reduce the circulation locally. A reduced circulation would prevent a normal circulatory response to cooling and might precipitate an ice burn. The pack may be left in position for 10–20 minutes.

3. **Ice water immersion:** Immersion is a technique in which the part to be treated is immersed in an ice solution. Unfortunately it is only practical to immerse certain areas such as hands, feet and elbows and it is subject to gravity-dependent positions.

   Preparation: The solution is made up of 50% ice and 50% water placed in a suitable container.

   Application: The patient immerses the part in the solution and keeps it in either for a single 10-minute session or for a series of shorter immersion until a cumulative total of 10 minutes has been reached. Often the patient experiences intense pain in the immersed area, sometimes severe enough to cause him to faint. He should therefore be suitably supported, and watched throughout the treatment.

4. **Ice massage:** This is the most common mode of application of cryotherapy as it does not require an ice machine. The freezer compartment of a domestic refrigerator is sufficient. It is used to deliver cold treatments to small, evenly shaped areas and often indicated with conditions requiring stretching.

   Preparation: A large block of ice, e.g. water frozen in a yoghurt pot or Styrofoam cup, has one end wrapped in a towel and the other end being left free. The patient is adequately exposed and supported. The patient may be able to administer self-treatment.

Application: The exposed end of the ice block is massaged in a circular manner over the small treatment area or longitudinal strokes (5–7 cm/sec) over the larger treatment area, by applying only minimal pressure to the part. The maximum time of application is 10 minutes or until the skin is numb to fine touch.

Ice-cube massage: This technique is particularly useful in the treatment of bedsores and pressure areas which are threatening to break down.

The ice is massaged gently on the skin surrounding the sore for about 2 minutes. The skin is then gently dried by dabbing or with warm airflow from a hair-dryer.

The ice application is repeated three or four times.

5. **Excitatory cold (quick ice):** The marked sensory stimulus of ice on the skin may be used to facilitate contraction of inhibited muscles.

   It is necessary first to find (myotome) of the inhibited muscle and then to find (dermatome) which has the same root supply. Once this has been done, the ice is stroked quickly three times over the dermatome and the skin is then dried.

   The sensory stimulus of cold passes via the peripheral nerve enters the spinal cord through the posterior horn of spinal cord.

   The anterior horn cells have many connections with these sensory fibers, and net result is thought to be, raising the level of excitation around the anterior horn cell.

   The increased excitation may be enough to supplement the patient's willed effort to make the muscle contract.

6. **Cold whirlpool:** Indicated in acute and subacute situations where exercise in cold environment is desired. Whirlpools are effective for treating large irregular shaped areas.

   Application: Fill appropriate size whirlpool with cold water and flaked ice with temperature at 60–80°F.

Patient submerges whole body or body part in the whirlpool after having turned on the turbine.

Once treatment is over, the patient removes himself from the whirlpool, dry off, and then turn off the turbine. The duration of treatment is 15–20 minutes.

7. **Cold compression units (cryo-cuffs):** These are the devices that alternately pump cold water at a temperature of 10°–25°C and air into a sleeve, that is wrapped around a patient's limb. Compression is also applied by intermittent inflation of the sleeve with air. These devices are most commonly used both acutely following injury and directly after surgery for the control of post-traumatic/postoperative inflammation and edema.

   Application: The part to be treated is exposed and put into a comfortable position. Apply the limb with stockinet before the sleeve is applied. The sleeve on application is wrapped around the area of treatment and the part is kept elevated. Cuffs come for specific areas of the body, i.e. shoulder, ankle, and knee. The temperature of chilled water which flow into sleeve from cooler is set between 10°–15°C. The cooling can be applied continuously as well as intermittently. As the cooler is raised pressure in the cuff is increased, providing a cooling effect with compression and elevation for post-surgery patients.

8. **Vapocoolant spray:** The technique of cooling in which volatile substances such as *ethyl chloride* or *fluoromethane*, etc. are sprayed directly on the area to be treated. This type of treatment is frequently applied in sports injury and for stretching of the tight muscles. Cooling is superficial without significant penetration and acts as a counterirritant to block pain.

   Application: The part to be treated is exposed and put into a comfortable position in the usual manner but in this technique an additional precaution is taken to protect the surrounding skin.

   Spraying technique: While the spray is applied the bottle is placed at a distance of about 45 cm from the skin and angled so that the spray hits the skin at an angle of about 30°. Two to five parallel sweeps of spray at a speed of approximately 10 cm per second along the direction of muscle fibers (proximal to distal) are generally applied. Static stretching can be incorporated as you spray.

9. **Contrast baths:** In contrast bath there is alternate immersion of the part in hot and cold water. Such a treatment causes considerable sensory stimulation due to activation of cutaneous hot and cold receptors. Generally used to treat subacute swelling.

   Preparation: Select two baths of a suitable size depending upon the size of the limb. Fill one bath with hot water maintained at a temperature of 40–45°C and the other with cold water maintained at a temperature of 10°–15°C. Expose the part to be treated and keep it in a comfortable position. Check the skin sensation for hot and cold.

   Application: If treatment is for pain relief, it is usual to start and end the treatment with hot water, whereas if treatment is for reducing edema, start and end the treatment with immersion in cold water.

   Place the limb in hot water for 3–4 minutes followed by immediate immersion in cold water for 1 minute (3:1 or 4:1 heat:cold ratios). Can reduce edema through "pumping" action (alternate vasodilatation and vasoconstriction).

   Repeat the treatment cycles for 3–4 times, so that the treatment time remains between 15 and 25 minutes.

10. **Cryostretch and cryokinetics:** *Cryostretch*—it is a combination of cold application and muscle stretching exercises. Ice reduces pain and muscle spasm and thereby facilitating better stretching of the tight structures. Begin with cryostretch then transition into cryokinetics.

Cryokinetics: It combines cryotherapy with exercises. Cold is applied for 12–20 minutes to produce numbness, following which the patient exercises the part for 3–5 minutes or till the sensation returned. At this point, ice is reapplied for 3–5 minutes until numbness returns. This process can be repeated five times. Exercises should be pain-free and progressive in intensity concentrating on both flexibility and strength.

LONG ANSWER QUESTIONS (15 MARKS)

Discuss the physiological effects of cold. Write the therapeutic uses and indications for same (Summer 2012).

OR

Describe physiological effects and uses of cold therapy. Write any five techniques of application of cold therapy and contraindication of cold therapy.

OR

What is latent heat of fusion and latent heat of vaporization? Discuss technique of application of ice any three. Write contraindications of ice treatment.

Latent heat: A specific amount of energy is required to change the solid form of a particular substance into a liquid or liquid into a gas. This energy is called latent heat.

- It is the energy required for (or released by) a change of state of matter.

Latent heat of fusion: In case of water, 1 gm of ice at 0°C requires 336 joules of energy to convert it to 1 gm of water at 0°C; this energy is called latent heat of fusion.

- Ice melting on the skin takes considerable energy (heat) from the skin, thus cooling it.

Latent heat of vaporization: 1 gm of water at 100°C requires 2268 Joules of energy to convert it to 1 gm of steam at 100°C; this energy is called latent heat of vaporization.

Practical application: Ice melting on the skin takes considerable energy (heat) from the skin, thus cooling it, whereas paraffin wax solidifying on the skin gives out considerable heat to the skin, thus warming it.

Techniques of ice application: Same as above.

Physiological effects and uses of cold therapy: Same as above.

Contraindications

The use of cryotherapy is contraindicated in the following conditions:

1. *Peripheral vascular diseases:* As cold application may cause vasoconstriction, along with an increase of blood

viscosity, it could reduce an already inadequate blood supply. Conditions such as arteriosclerosis and other peripheral vascular disorders, where there is an impairment of blood circulation over a particular area are contraindicated. In general, do not use cold over areas of compromised circulation.

2. *Vasospastic disorders:* The vasospasm in diseases such as Raynaud should not be treated with cryotherapy, as cold may further induce vasoconstriction thereby impairing circulation.

3. *Cardiac conditions:* Caution should be taken when treating patients with cardiac disease such as myocardial infarct. As the initial shock of ice application may cause marked drop in blood pressure, thus causing an increase in heart rate—A weak heart may not be able to meet this demand.

   The left shoulder and the heart have the same sympathetic nerve supply and ice applied to the left shoulder may cause an overflow of excitatory impulses to the heart via these sympathetic nerves. Therefore, ice to the left shoulder should be avoided in patients with cardiac disease.

4. *Peripheral nerve injuries:* Blood vessels in the area supplied by a severed peripheral nerve lose their normal response to cooling and the part may get very cold.

   Cryotherapy should not be applied directly over a regenerating peripheral nerve, as local vasoconstriction may reduce blood supply to the peripheral nerves and may cause its further damage.

5. *Cold sensitivity (urticaria):* Following the application of ice, some patients develop bumps on the skin which looks like a nettle rash and itches, due to release of histamine from the mast cells.

6. *Psychological factor:* The patients having fear of cold, particularly the elderly, may react adversely. If the therapist cannot persuade or demonstrate to the patient that ice will be beneficial then it might be better not to use it.

WHIRLPOOL BATH

A whirlpool bath is a tank that contains water with a turbine in it to produce movement of water through agitation and aeration, making it enables to assist or resist movements of the distal parts of the extremities or the whole extremity and the lower trunk (Fig. 11.9).

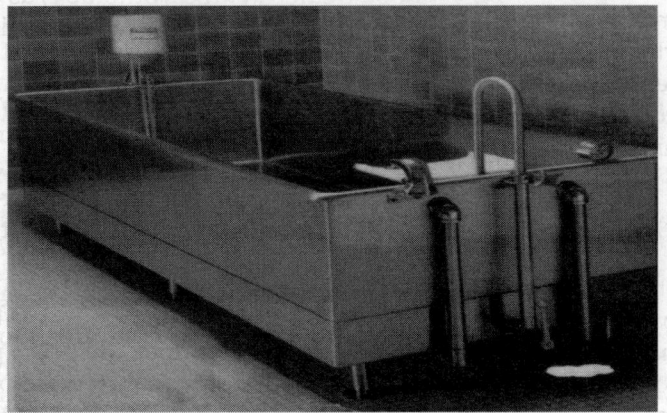

Fig. 11.9: The whirlpool bath

The tank is usually made of stainless steel. The shapes and sizes of the tanks are also variable. The turbine of the whirlpool is composed of a motor bracketed securely to the side of the whirlpool, with pipes for water and air circulation suspended in the water.

The height and direction of the turbine determines the effect. There is a mixing tap to allow any desired water temperature; a temperature of 36–41°C are usually employed, but for the treatment of acutely inflamed structures, a temperature of 0°–26°C (cold whirlpool) is used.

TECHNIQUE OF APPLICATION

The tank is filled with water and the required temperature is selected using the thermostat. If required an antimicrobial agent is added to water, particularly for the treatment of open wounds.

The patient is prepared as per any heat/cold treatments. No clothing should be allowed to enter into the water, as it may be sucked into the turbine. Position the patient comfortably with the affected area immersed in water.

Adjust the direction and aeration of the turbine, as per the effect required. Turn on the turbine and tell the patient to exercise the affected part if treatment is directed for joint stiffness or edema without acute inflammation.

Treatment time is usually confined to 10–30 minutes, though shorter period may be indicated for wound debridement. At the end of treatment, the limb should be kept out of water, thoroughly checked and is covered by a dry sheet to avoid chilling.

CONTRAST BATH

Contrast baths are an alternative method of applying heat with a certain amount of cold to aid the normal body temperature regulating mechanism. There is alternate immersion of the part in hot and cold water. This treatment helps to modulate pain, as the strong sensory stimulation does the same by the pain gate mechanism and it also reduces local edema by the alternate vasoconstriction and vasodilatation.

METHODS OF APPLICATION

Select two baths of a suitable size depending upon the size of the part to be treated. Fill one bath with hot water maintained at a temperature of 40°–45°C and the other with cold water maintained at a temperature of 15°–20°C.

Expose the part to be treated and remove the ornament and check the skin sensation for hot and cold.

Check for any other contraindications like defective arterial blood supply, open wounds, etc.

If the treatment is for pain relief, it is usual to start and end the treatment with hot water, whereas if the treatment is for reducing edema, start and end the treatment with immersion in cold water.

Place the limb in hot water for 3–4 minutes followed by immediate immersion in cold water for 1 minute. Repeat the treatment cycles for 3–4 times, so that the treatment time remains within 15–25 minutes.

During treatment maintain the hot and cold water at a constant temperature. Check the skin after treatment. The skin may show mild erythema after the treatment.

PELOIDS

Peloids (7 Marks)

The term *peloid* refers to the pulp of a substance. The most common peloids are made of peat, lake mud, sea mud, or plant material. For more than 200 years in Europe, peloid packs and baths using peat have been used for medicinal purposes.

Types of mud or peloids used in treatment are of the following types:

a. **Mineral mud or fango:** This type consists essentially of volcanic ashes found near lakes. It contains sulfur, iron, silicates and radioactive material.

b. **Mineral sea mud:** This type consists of remains of sea life. It is found along the shores of waterways.

c. **Organic moor or peat mud:** It consists of decaying or decomposed vegetable matter as from rots, leaves. This type of mud is found in a crude form and must be processed before being used for packs and baths.

Methods of Application

- **For a peloid peat pack treatment:** Peloids in a small cotton bag are heated at the temperature of 45°–48°C and are placed on the part of the body to be treated. If water is used in a mixture with mud or peat, the mixture is spread evenly on the cloth and tested for the desired temperature. Once the temperature is tested it is placed on the affected area and molded around the part covered with plastic. A terry towel is applied over the top and left for 20 minutes. Remove the bag, clean the area by spraying water and rewrap the part until patient cool down.
- **For the medicinal peat bath:** A bath is filled 10 inches from the top with water at a temperature of 105°–113°F. The

duration and temperature of the bath depend on the condition being treated. Peat is added to the bath, and the patient enters the water slowly.

The patient remains submerged below the neck for 8–20 minutes, and is then helped from the tub and onto a table covered in a clean sheet. Two or three wool blankets are wrapped around the patient's body. The patient remains wrapped for about 30 minutes to stimulate perspiration.

Patients are advised not to shower for 12 hours after a peat bath to allow the peat additives to continue to be absorbed.

Indications of Mud Baths and Packs

Chronic inflammatory joint conditions causing joint pain: Osteoarthritis, rheumatoid arthritis, chronic back pain (lumbago, sciatica), chronic post-traumatic stiffness, strains, sprains, neuritis (peripheral) due to diabetes, gout, neuralgia, pain relief, fibromyalgia.

Contraindications of Peloids Application

Acute inflammation, sensitive skin, infection wounds, heart disease (high BP, circulatory insufficiency), respiratory disease, cancer.

Disadvantages of Peloids

Difficulty in storing and heating the mud in a special container. Not practical for inpatients treatments as rather messy.

Difficulty in supplying the mud if the department is located in geographical areas that are not producing the mud.

Cross infection risks and not easy disposal of the mud.

Therefore, it appears that peloids are more often used in spa or health centers than in hospital settings.

ELECTRICAL HEATING PADS

Electrical Heating Pads (7 Marks)

A method of applying low-level heat over a long time has been available for years in the form of electric heating pads. It can be a square or in any other shape-like the cervical pads, that vary from small pads about 30 by 30 cm to electric blankets. It contains series of electrical wires that is covered by suitable fabric and plastic pouch. These wires are connected to a small box outside that serves as a thermostat that has an electrical plug extending from it. The fabric cover should be put over the pouch to protect from skin burns.

These pads are particularly useful for treatment at home and for producing muscle relaxation prior to other treatments such as exercises or mobilization.

Advantages

1. Readily available for purchase at a reasonable cost for long-term use.
2. A convenient method of at-home heat application to be used.
3. Provide a comfortable, dry heat sensation.

Disadvantages

1. Can cause skin and subcutaneous tissue burns if the patient falls asleep during treatment.
2. Patient must be near an electrical outlet during use.
3. Patient cannot exercise while applying the pad.

Indications: General indications for electric heating pads include pain, muscle spasm, contracture, tension myalgia, bursitis, tenosynovitis, fibrositis, fibromyalgia.

Contraindications: General contraindications include: Acute inflammation, trauma, hemorrhage, bleeding disorders, temperature insensitivity such as the peripheral neuropathy in diabetic patients, poor thermal regulation, malignancy, edema, ischemia, atrophic skin, scar tissue.

HOT COMPRESSES

Hot Compresses (7 Marks)

Hot local compresses are primarily for home use and are not practical for clinical use. There is greater heat loss than with hydrocollator packs, and therefore the compresses have to be changed constantly.

Technique of Application of Hot Compresses

- Equipment required: Turkish towel, strips of woolen blanket or of any absorbent material, hot water at a temperature of 40° to 42°C or hot towel machine, timer.
- Position the patient comfortably with the part to be treated fully supported. Check the skin area to be treated.
- Place a large towel in a basin with the free ends hanging out. Place a smaller towel inside the large towel. Pour hot water onto the towels and wring them out. Make sure the towels are thoroughly wet. Apply the towels to the desired area.
- To maintain constant heat, cover the compress with a hot water bottle, or use and infrared lamp, or wrap in a blanket. Apply the compress for 20 minutes, changing every 5 minutes.
- Check the skin after the removal of the hot compress.

Indications and contraindications: If hydrocollator packs are not available, hot compresses can be used as an alternative. See hydrocollator packs for indications and contraindications.

Precautions in Applying Compresses

- Make sure that the towels are wrung out properly. Apply a compress which is only as hot as the patient can bear.
- If the compress is too hot, remove quickly; wipe any excess moisture from the skin and reapply.
- In treating children, tolerance should be built up gradually during the first application to prevent a fear reaction by the child.
- Fit the compress to the contour of the part to prevent air from entering and cooling the compress.
- Have fluids ready to minimize dehydration.

FLUIDOTHERAPY

Fluidotherapy (7 Marks)

- Despite the name, it does not use fluid to heat the tissues. This is a dry-heating modality that consists of cellulose particles circulated by hot air. Because this unit uses dry heat transferred by convection in a suspended airstream, patients can tolerate a much higher temperature than they would with either paraffin wax or moist heat (Fig. 11.10). However, this is still a superficial heat therapy.

- Recommended temperature varies by body part and patient tolerance, with a range of 110° to 125°F (43°–53°C). Maximum temperature rise occurs after 15 minutes of treatment and total treatment duration is 15–20 minutes.

- Effects of fluidotherapy include general heating effects, plus micromassage, levitation, and stimulation. Exercise during the treatment can help increase the range of motion and ability to perform.

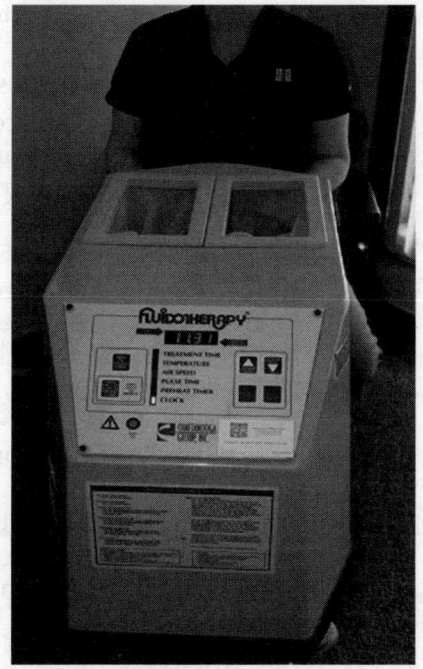

Fig. 11.10: Fluidotherapy unit

Indications and Contraindications

Indications and contraindications are the same as other heating modalities.

Application procedures

Step 1: The patient's extremity is inserted into an enclosed port location either at the side or top of the unit.

Step 2: Temperature of the modality is set between 110° and 125°F.

Step 3: Particle agitation/blower intensity should be set at the patient comfort level.

Post-treatment procedures: Check the patient's skin following treatment for any adverse reaction that may have occurred. Have the patient monitor their symptoms later in the day for any increased stiffness, achiness, or pain.

Testing of Apparatus

ELECTRICAL MUSCLE STIMULATOR

Knobs

Intensity knob: The intensity of current that is passed to the patient is regulated by rheostat.

Surge interval: It is the interval between the two pulses or contractions.

Surge duration: It is the time or duration for which the contraction lasts.

Millisecond duration: It is a duration for interrupted galvanic current. It is marked from 0.01 to 300.

Frequency: It is the number of cycles per second. It is marked from 1 to 100.

Timer: It is used to set the time for which the machine is to be used.

Mains: It indicates that the machine is working.

Output: Black output is for cathode and red output is for anode.

Materials Required

Cotton: It is used to clean the area to be tested.

Mackintosh: It is a non-conducting material and the part to be tested is placed on it.

Bowl: Bowl with tap water which is used to clean the part to be treated.

Tester: It is used to check the mains supply.

Lint pad: It is made up of cotton fabric which is 6–8 folds.

Micropore: It is used to fix the electrodes.

Electrode gel: It acts as a medium for the passage of current.

Electrodes: Used to give output of the muscle stimulator (metal plate, carbon rubber, pen electrode).

Preparation of Apparatus

The testing of mains and apparatus is done with the help of a tester.

The active electrode may be a disc electrode/pen electrode. A flat plate electrode with lint pad is used as an indifferent electrode to complete the circuit.

The lint pad consists of at least 6–8 folds so that they are thick enough to make contact with tissues and to absorb any chemicals which might be formed. They must be folded evenly with no creases or there shall be uneven distribution of current and they can cause discomfort.

The lint pad covering the plate electrode is soaked in warm 1% saline water since it reduces the skin resistance. Electrodes should be ½ inch smaller than the lint pad to reduce the danger of their coming in contact with the skin and causing discomfort/damage. Corner of the electrode should be rounded as point may become bent and dig into the pad thus causing concentration of current.

Preparation of the Part

The resistance of the skin is reduced by washing with soap and water to remove the natural oil.

Procedure

Connect the plug to the 3-pin wall socket. Turn all the knobs to zero, switch on the power supply and see if the pilot lamp is glowing. This confirms that the machine is on.

The active electrode (pen electrode) is connected to the positive terminal colored red and the passive electrode to the negative terminal colored black. The therapist tests the apparatus by attaching the electrodes to the terminals, holding the two electrodes in a moistened hand, turning up the current until a mild prickling sensation is experienced and a muscle contraction is produced. This confirms that the machine is working. After which all the knobs are turned to zero, the machine is switched off and the electrodes are removed (Figs 12.1 and 12.2).

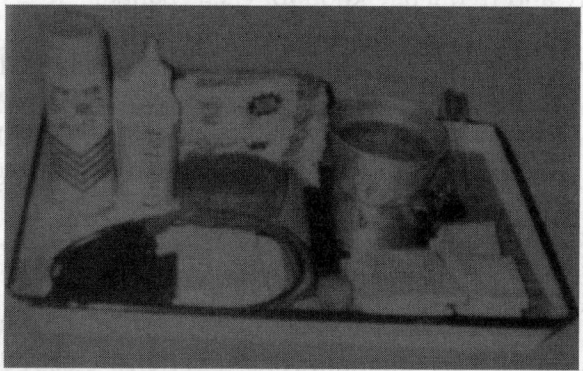

Fig. 12.1: Treatment tray

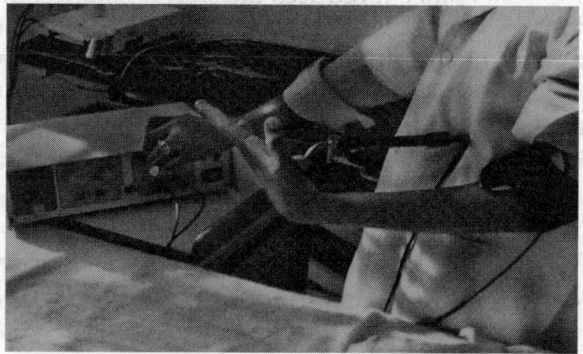

Fig. 12.2: Testing of the electrical muscle stimulator

TRANSCUTANEOUS ELECTRICAL NERVE STIMULATOR

Knobs

Intensity knob: It is the intensity of current that is passed to the patient. It is regulated by rheostat.

Frequency: It is the number of cycles per second. It is marked from 1 to 100.

Timer: It is used to set the time for which the machine is to be used.

Output: They are used to attach the electrodes into them. It may have two channels or four channels and there is separate intensity and frequency knob for each channel.

Materials Required

Bowl of water: Bowl with tap water which is used to clean the part to be treated.

Mackintosh: It is a non-conducting material and the part to be tested is placed on it.

Velcro strap: It is used to fix the electrodes.

Cotton: It is used to clean the area tested

Electrode gel: It acts as a medium for passage of current.

Electrodes: Each channel consists of two electrodes with two different colors (e.g. red for anode and black for cathode).

Preparation of Apparatus

The testing of mains and apparatus is done with the help of a tester.

Check the insulation of the wire.

Check that all the knobs are at zero before starting the treatment.

Preparation of the Part

The resistance of the skin is reduced by washing with soap and water to remove the natural oil.

Procedure

Connect the plug to the 3-pin wall socket. Turn all the knobs to zero, switch on the power and see if the pilot lamp is glowing. This confirms that the machine is on.

The operator tests the apparatus by attaching the electrodes to the terminals holding the two electrodes in a moistened hand, turning up the current gradually until a mild prickling sensation is experienced. This confirms that the machine is working.

After which all the knobs are turned to zero, the machine is switched off and the electrodes are removed.

INTERFERENTIAL THERAPY

Knobs

Timer: It is used to set the time for which the machine is used for testing.

Intensity: It is used to regulate the amount of current applied to the patient.

Balance: It is used to regulate the intensity in either of the electrodes.

Beat frequency: It is the difference between the frequencies of the two interfering current.

It ranges from 0 to 150 scan, 80 to 150 scan, 0 to 10 scan, 0 to 150 continuous.

Frequency: It ranges from 2 to 4 KHz.

Sweep pattern: There are three patterns—rectangular, triangular and trapezoidal.

Treatment mode: There are three treatment modes—2-pole, 4-pole and 4-pole vector.

Start/stop: It is used to on/off the machine.

Materials Required

Bowl of water: Bowl with tap water which is used to clean the part to be treated.

Mackintosh: It is a non-conducting material and the part to be tested is placed on it.

Micropore: It is used to fix the electrodes.

Cotton: It is used to clean the area tested

Electrode gel: It acts as a medium for passage of current.

Electrodes: A channel consists of two electrodes with two different colors (red and blue).

Lint pad: Used to prevent the accumulation of chemicals in the tissues to prevent chemical burn.

Types of Electrodes

Plate electrodes: These are made up of conducting rubbers which are comfortable and long lasting.

Vacuum electrodes: These are rubber suction cups connected to the machine capable of producing vacuum. They are really plate electrode kept in position by vacuum instead of bandaging.

Methods of placing electrodes

1. *Two-pole method:* In this method only 2 electrodes are used either red channel or black channel electrodes. Here continuous beat frequency is used and premodulated interference is produced within the machine.
2. *Four-pole method:* Four electrodes are used by placing one channel of electrodes diagonally opposite to each other. The area covered is minimum since electric field is constant.
3. *Four-pole vector:* In this method four electrodes are placed on the area covered which is large as electric field is rotating in alternating pattern.

Preparation of Apparatus

The testing of mains and apparatus is done with the help of a tester.

- Check the insulation of the wire.
- Check whether all the knobs are at zero.
- Check whether fuse is present in the apparatus that is not blown out.

Preparation of the Part

Expose the part to be tested. The resistance of the skin is reduced by washing with soap and water to remove the natural oil. The electrodes are placed in such a way that they must not contact each other. If two pole method is used then only one channel of electrodes are placed side by side with some gap between them.

If four-pole method or four-pole vector method is used then two channels of electrode are placed diagonally to each other. The crossing point of two currents is above the part to be tested.

One hand is placed over the electrodes and with the other hand intensity knob is turned.

Procedure

Switch on the machine. Set the parameters such as frequency, sweep pattern, mode, etc.

Place the electrode on the part to be tested according to the treatment mode chosen. Gradually increase the intensity until the therapist feels the tingling sensation. This ensures that the machine is working properly. After the testing turn the knob to zero and switch off the machine (Fig. 12.3).

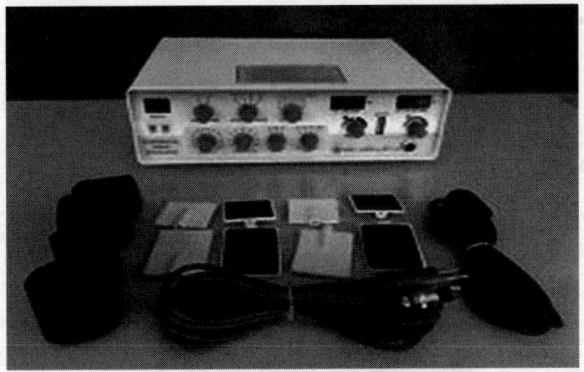

Fig. 12.3: Interferential therapy machine

SHORT WAVE DIATHERMY

Knobs

Mains: It is red pilot which indicates if the machine is on/off.

Voltage knob: Used to set the voltage.

Power knob: Used to set the power of the machine.

Tuning knob: Match the frequency of the oscillator/machine circuit and the resonator/patient circuit.

Types of Electrodes

There are various types of electrodes. Electrodes could be pad electrode, plate electrode and disc electrode. Each electrode consists of a metal plate surrounded by some form of insulating material.

1. *Pad electrode:* Thin malleable metal plate covered with a rubber pad. It has an advantage to get moulded according to the body part.

2. *Malleable/flexible plate electrode:* It consists of a thick rigid metal plate coated with a thin layer of rubber insulating material made up of rubber or plastic.

3. *Disc electrode:* These are having a plastic transparent cover within which a metal plate is present. These electrodes are commonly circular in shape (Fig. 12.4).

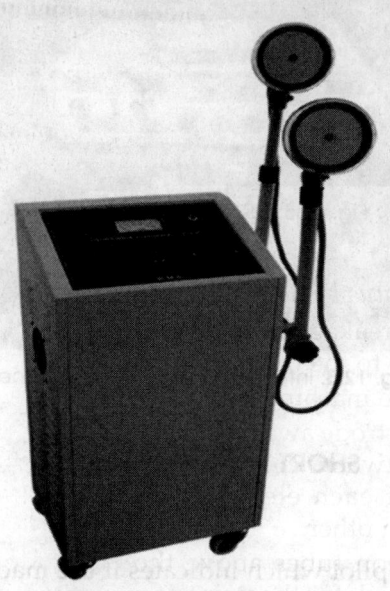

Fig. 12.4: SWD with disc electrodes

Procedure

Testing of apparatus by hand

- Check any breakage in the circuit by using tester.
- Connect the electrode to the outlet.
- Switch on the machine.
- Place the electrode away from each other on a stable surface.

- Distance between the electrodes is equal to the sum of thickness of each electrode.
- Make sure cables are not crossing each other.
- Place your hand over the electrode and tune the machine.
- Check for the point of maximum deflection and feel the heat (Fig. 12.5).

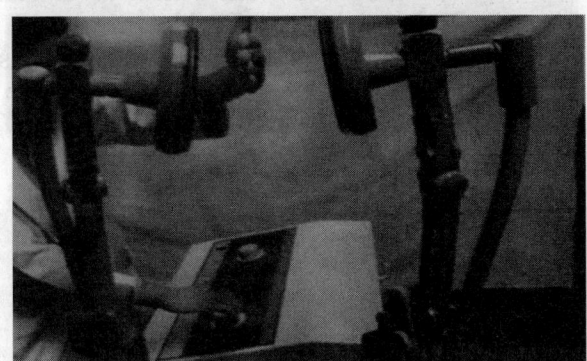

Fig. 12.5: Testing of SWD by hand

Testing of apparatus by neon tube
- Check any breakage in the circuit by using tester. Connect the electrode to the outlet.
- Switch on the machine.
- Place the electrode away from each other on a stable surface. Distance between the electrodes is equal to the sum of thickness of each electrode. Make sure cables are not crossing each other.
- Place the neon tubes above the electrodes and tune the machine. Check for the point of maximum deflection. If the neon tube is glowing the apparatus is working (Fig. 12.6).

ULTRASOUND THERAPY

Ultrasound refers to the mechanical vibrations which are essentially the same as sound waves, but has a frequency higher than audible frequency limit, i.e. frequency >20,000 Hz (Figs 12.7 and 12.8).

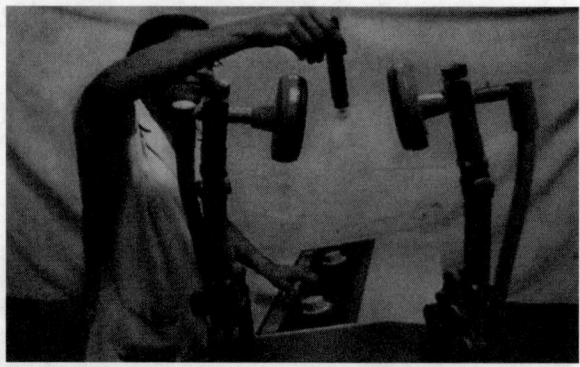

Fig. 12.6: Testing of SWD with neon lamp

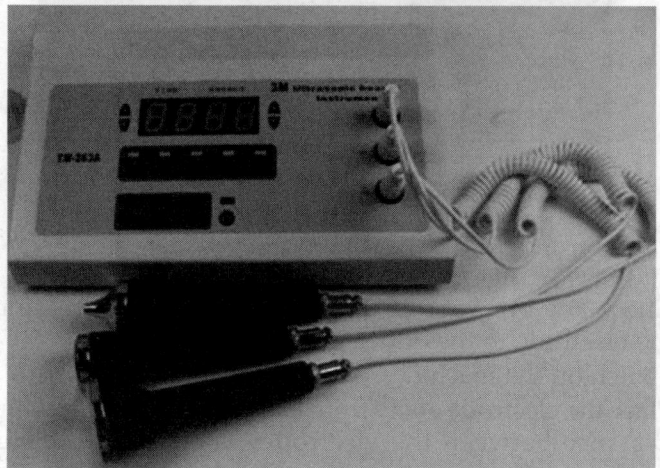

Fig. 12.7: Therapeutic ultrasound

Knobs

Timer: It is the time adjustment for which the machine is kept on.

Intensity knob: This indicates the power output of the machine (W/cm^2).

Modes: It involves either continuous or pulsed mode.

Pilot lamp (red): This indicates the machine is on.

On/off switch: Used to switch on/off the machine.

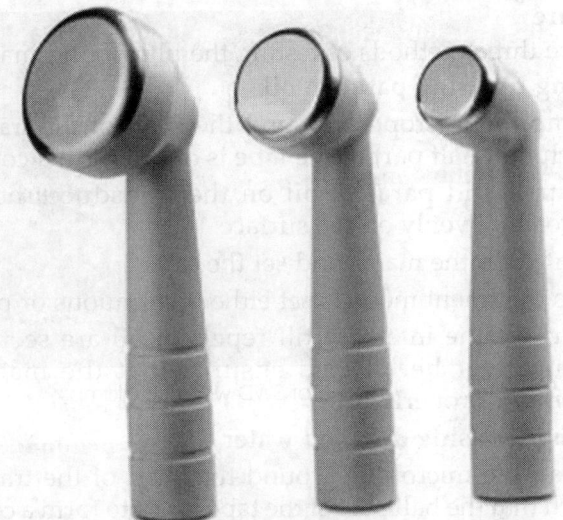

Fig. 12.8: Ultrasound treatment head

Materials Required

1. Liquid paraffin oil　2. Distilled water　3. Cotton
4. Bowl　　　　　　　5. Metal reflector　6. Micropore

Preparation of Part

The therapist should be comfortably seated with arm supported and the part should be exposed. The couplant should be applied to the skin surface. The therapist ensures that close contact, appropriate movement and correct angle of the transducer are maintained at all times. The treatment head is placed on the skin before output is turned on.

Preparation of Machine

The testing of mains and apparatus is done with the help of a tester.

- Check the insulation of the wire.
- Check that all the knobs are at zero.
- Check the connection of transducer with a machine.

Procedure

There are three methods of testing the ultrasound machine:

1. Testing by using paraffin oil

- Wrap the micropore around the head of the transducer such that half part of the tape is out to form a covering.
- Pour liquid paraffin oil on the transducer head and spread it evenly on the surface.
- Switch on the mains and set the time.
- The treatment mode is set either continuous or pulsed.
- Increase the intensity till repels of oil are seen on the transducer head. This ensures that the machine is working properly.

2. Testing by using distilled water

- Wrap the micropore around the head of the transducer such that the half part of the tape is out to form a covering.
- Pour the distilled water on the transducer head and spread it evenly on the surface.
- Switch on the mains and set the time.
- The treatment mode is set either continuous or pulsed.
- Increase the intensity till repels of water are seen on the transducer head. This ensures that the machine is working properly.

3. Testing underwater

- Take a bowl filled with distilled water. Place a metal reflector inside the bowl at an angle of 45° with the bowl.
- Immerse the head of the transducer inside the bowl.
- Turn on the machine and set the timer.
- The treatment mode is set either continuous or pulsed.
- Increase the intensity till repels are seen on the surface near the reflector. This ensures that the machine is working properly.

INFRARED RADIATION (IR) LAMP

Infrared radiation is electromagnetic energy invisible to human eye, having wavelength between 760 and 1 mm that lies within visible light and microwave radiation (Fig. 12.9).

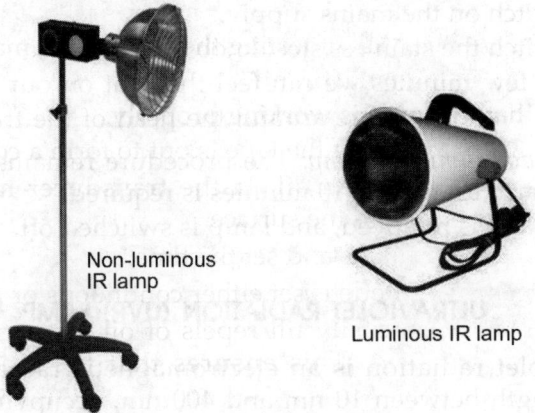

Non-luminous
IR lamp

Luminous IR lamp

Fig. 12.9: Types of IR lamp

Preparation of Lamp

The lamp is positioned to allow the radiations to strike the skin at a right angle, to facilitate maximum absorption of the rays. The distance of the lamp from the patient should be 50–75 cm depending upon the output of the generator.

When there is acute inflammation or recent injury, the sedative effect of the rays obtained from non-luminous generator is more effective for relieving pain. For lesions of a more chronic type, a luminous generator is chosen.

If the output is to be maximizing the non-luminous generator must be switch on for 10 minutes and the luminous generator for few minutes before use.

Preparation of Patient

The subject is positioned comfortably.

The clothing is removed and the skin is checked for its sensation against heat and cold.

The eyes are shielded if they are likely to be irradiated in order to prevent drying of the surface.

Procedure

Testing of machine

With luminous lamp: Place your dorsal aspect of hand beneath the lamp at the distance of 50–70 cm.

- Switch on the mains supply.
- Switch the stainless steel knob to IR.

After few minutes we can feel the heat on our hand, this ensures that the lamp is working properly.

With non-luminous lamp: The procedure remains the same just a warm up time of 10 minutes is required.

The hand is removed, and lamp is switched off.

ULTRAVIOLET RADIATION (UVR) LAMP

Ultraviolet radiation is an electromagnetic radiation with wavelength between 10 nm and 400 nm, occupying a place between X-ray and visible light in the electromagnetic spectrum.

The ultraviolet spectrum is further subdivided into three regions:

1. UVA: 400–315 nm
2. UVB: 315–280 nm
3. UVC: 280–100 nm

Testing of UVR Lamp

Preparation of the part: The part is washed to remove any dust or grease by soap and soaked with a towel to remove any moisturizer. A thin film of petroleum jelly can be applied over dorsum of the hand.

The rest of the body which does not need exposure should be covered with appropriate clothing. The eyes need to be protected by cotton wool or protective goggles.

Preparation of the lamp: The lamp should be placed at 90° to the part to be tested.

It should be kept at the distance of 50–75 cm from the part to be tested.

Procedure

After testing of mains supply and casing of the lamp with tester, switch on the mains supply.

Switch on the stainless steel knob to UVR. After 5 minutes heat is felt if dorsal aspect of the hand is placed beneath the lamp at specified distance or bright glowing of the lamp can be seen which ensures that the lamp is working properly.

Switch off the lamp and then the mains.

LASER

The popularly used term LASER is an acronym for light amplification by stimulated emission of radiation.

Low intensity laser therapy or low laser therapy is the therapeutic application of relatively low output (<500 mW) lasers for the treatment of musculoskeletal disorders and injuries at dosages (usually <35 J/cm^2), generally considered to be too low to effect any detectable heating of the irradiated tissues (Figs 12.10 and 12.11).

Testing of Laser Machine

Preparation of the part
- The part is supported in such a way that any pressure of the laser applicator does not cause movement or discomfort.
- The surface of the skin to be tested is cleaned with an alcohol wipe, in order to remove any material formed on the surface that might absorb or scatter the radiation.
- The physiotherapist should wear protective goggles.

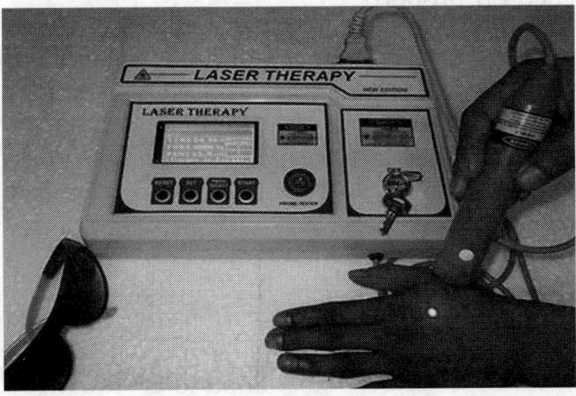

Fig. 12.10: Laser therapy unit

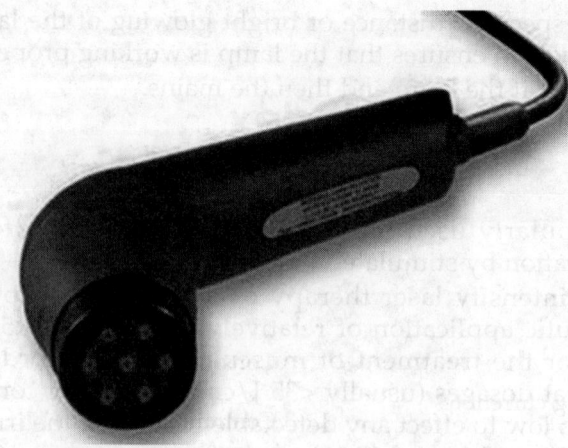

Fig. 12.11: Cluster probe of laser

Procedure
- The laser probe is selected depending upon the nature and size of the lesion.
- Place the laser generator probe towards the wall.
- Switch on the machine.
- Set the parameters such as continuous or pulse, power, etc.
- Look for the laser beam on the wall.
- Red pencil-like point on the wall can be seen. This ensures that the machine is working properly. The device is switched off properly.

Index